Alkaline Diet For Disease Prevention

The Ultimate Guide to Eat Healthy, Fight Inflammation, Lose Weight and Fight Cronic Disease

Hilda Shilling

The reproduction, transmission, and duplication of any of the content found herein, including any specific or extended information, will be done as an illegal act regardless of the end form the information ultimately takes. This includes copied versions of the work, both physical, digital, and audio unless express consent of the Publisher is provided beforehand. Any additional rights reserved.

Furthermore, the information that can be found within the pages described forthwith shall be considered both accurate and truthful when it comes to the recounting of facts. As such, any use, correct or incorrect, of the provided information will render the Publisher free of responsibility as to the actions taken outside of their direct purview. Regardless, there are zero scenarios where the original author or the Publisher can be deemed liable in any fashion for any damages or hardships that may result from any of the information discussed herein.

Additionally, the information in the following pages is intended only for informational purposes and should thus be thought of as universal. As befitting its nature, it is presented without assurance regarding its prolonged validity or interim quality. Trademarks that are mentioned are done without written consent and can in no way be considered an endorsement from the trademark holder.

Chapter One

Alkaline Diet Basics

The human body is a marvelous entity which works best when the proper nutrition is provided. How we consume impacts our quality of life generally, and how our bodies work. This may be tough in today's culture to supply the body with the correct nutrients, since prepared refined products are too cheap and readily accessible. Nevertheless, all of these products throw off the equilibrium of our bodies by not supplying adequate nutrients and adversely impacting our pH.

Recent science is showing that our body's acidity or alkalinity has a lot to do with our wellbeing and wellness. Creating your diet around alkaline food products is proving helpful for your overall health. Thankfully, it is simple to establish an alkaline diet particularly with whole, plant-based proteins

The body works very hard to control pH every day. This achieves this for two of our most essential filter organs: the lungs and the kidneys. Of starters, the exertion of muscles produces lactic acid, and extra carbon dioxide causes an acidic atmosphere in the blood, affecting all of the body functions. The kidneys and lungs function to eliminate this natural acid on a daily basis; however, you may increase the immediate risk of acidosis by adding foods which contribute to the acid imbalance. Acidosis is a disease triggered by a excess of acid in the body.

The condition has two forms, respiratory and biochemical, which all result in exhaustion, sleeplessness, lack of focus, and shortness of breath. Researchers are now showing that eating a diet rich in foods that support alkalinity with high mineral and nutrient concentrations will help the kidneys and lungs enter a mildly alkaline condition that helps the body to survive.

What Is The Alkaline Diet

Through removing excess acid the human body is built to retain a closely controlled pH balance. The Traditional American Diet primarily relies on items such as white bread, starch, agricultural products, and alcohol. Our bodies can tolerate both of these products, so when we overeat acidifying things and consume not enough of the products that help the capacity of our body to neutralize the acid, we are imbalanced. At times the body is unable to remove enough acid to achieve an acceptable balance. Some researchers believe it is this disparity that contributes to different diseases and illnesses.

The Alkaline Diet highlights foods which promote blood and urine alkalinity. These involve berries, vegetables and some whole grains. This diet combines the acidification of proteins with the alkalization of products, and the body functions easier.

Well living and treating the body with the love it earns implies providing it with the nutrients it requires. Our body regulates pH with our kidneys and lungs, and by maintaining these two organs safe we can help get rid of extra acid and survive on our bodies. Kidneys, like every other muscle, survive on a pure mineral mixture. Potassium, magnesium, chloride are three main minerals that allow our kidneys to function at their best, which in the modern diet, unfortunately, are few and far between.

Both of these things find it impossible for the body to absorb and provide too little nutrients. It hurts the kidneys, and the entire body. Happily, it's very straightforward to build a diet that encourages alkalinity. Foods that contain high nutrient amounts and minerals that grow on the liver, lungs, and other organs include green leafy plants, fresh fruits, and plant-based protein sources. When introducing one of those things to your diet, you will help your kidneys do their job to get rid of extra acid in your body.

Choosing a consistently balanced diet will help the kidneys and lungs maintain the optimal pH of only marginally alkaline at 7.4 for the body. You will guarantee that your body has the nutrients it requires to help you lead a balanced and vibrant life by adding nutrient-dense plants, new fruits and a plant-based protein.

What Is Ph

The pH scale is used to assess how acidic, normal, or neutral water dependent mixtures are used.

A material that is stable is neither acidic, nor basic. The pH meter, varying from 0 to 14, tests exactly how acidic or basic a material is. Higher numbers indicate a material is either alkaline (the "normal" and "alkaline" say the same thing for our purposes) or neutral, whereas lower numbers imply the material is more acidic.

This is neutral with a pH of 7.

A pH of about 7 is acidic.

This is alkaline with a pH higher than 7.

Many items used in the Alkaline Diet can have an acidic pH (like lemons), but the impact on the body is alkalizing. Yeah, you can't just know whether to consume a certain food by simply gazing at the pH point.

The Difference Between Acidic Waste and Acidic Foods

Acidic products and acidic diets have different body effects. Acid pollution is destructive — it sucks away nutrients and tissue becomes inflamed. At the other side, sour-tasting (acidic) foods provide the body with the acid which it uses to digest protein.

The many societies who follow what the "experts" say are overwhelmingly acidic diets are evidence who acidic food products do not affect the pH component of the body, or trigger degenerative disease. But their durability is uncertain. One illustration is the macrobiotic diet Dr. Sagen Ishizuka created in the latter half of the 19th century to treat his kidney failure which Western medicine had failed to achieve. Because it is based on the principle of combining opposites — yin (acid) and yang (alkaline)—the macrobiotic diet's dietary cornerstone is brown rice, which includes a large degree of acid-forming phosphorous.

In the 1930s, Dr. Weston Price, an American dentist, travelled to Asia, the outback of Australia and the Arctic to research the connection between food and wellbeing in the communities of those countries, who mostly practiced their ancestors 'ancestral diets. He discovered that many of the communities who adopted a grain-based diet rich in acid-forming phosphorous were in healthy, safe wellbeing.

A diet rich in alkaline minerals does not seem to be appropriate either for health preservation or for usual 7.4 alkaline blood plasma pH. Standardizing acid-alkaline blood pH by consuming more products in alkaline-forming minerals than acidic ones would not be the foundation for a diet for two more reasons: First, clusters of acidic, radioactive waste do not generally raise blood acid rates in various areas of the body.

This is unlikely that regulating the pH of blood by feeding will result in any inroads into amounts of acidic waste found far from large blood sources. Second, the amount of enzymes, bile, hydrochloric acid, and other metabolites that the body creates for nutritional breakdown is not calculated by the pH in the blood, but by the specific food tastes and protein that preserved the ancestors of the adult for thousands of years.

Acidic Foods That Are Alkalizing

You may ask how certain things outside the body may be acidic but have alkalising results when consumed. The response lies in the food's "fire" quality until burned. If a meal gets burned — this is something that food science perform in a regulated environment; your bbq is unlikely to produce trustworthy outcomes, no matter how badly your burgers get burned — if the resultant ash content becomes more alkaline than acid, it's called an alkalizing product. The explanation is that it undergoes oxidation as our body digests food, which is close to fire, and the effect is what decides whether the finished product becomes alkaline or acidic.

Acid- Foods To Restrict

You'll want to restrict all animal items (meat, dairy, fish and eggs) on the Alkaline Diet. Alcohol, caffeine and green tea are often discouraged, because they are strongly acidic. Similarly, we can stop processed sugars of some sort. And, considering that certain grains have an acidifying impact on the body, they can also be prevented.

A more detailed collection of acid- products labeled "No Go" continues to stop.

Acidifying legumes, seeds, and milks

- Rice milk
- Soy beans
- Soy milk
- Unsprouted beans

Acidifying Fats and Oils

- Avocado oil
- Butter
- Canola oil
- Corn oil
- Flax oil
- Hemp oil
- Lard
- Olive oil
- Safflower oil
- Sunflower oil

Acidifying Fruits

- Blueberries
- Canned or glazed fruits
- Cranberries
- Currants

Acidifying Grains and Grain Products

- Amaranth
- Barley
- Bran, oat
- Bran, wheat
- Bread
- Corn
- Cornstarch
- Crackers, soda
- Flour, wheat
- Flour, white
- Hemp seed flour
- Kamut
- Noodles
- Oatmeal
- Oats, rolled
- Pasta
- Rice cakes
- Rice, white

- Rye

- Spelt

- Wheat

- Wheat germ

Acidifying Nuts and Butters

- Cashews

- Legumes

- Peanut butter

- Peanuts

- Pecans

- Tahini

- Walnuts

Acidifying Sweeteners

- Carob

- Corn syrup

- Sugar

Acidifying Vegetables

- Corn

- Lentils

- Olives

All Alcohol

- Beer
- Hard liquor
- Spirits
- Wine

All Animal Protein

- Beef
- Eggs
- Fish
- Lamb
- Organ meats
- Pork
- Poultry
- Rabbit
- Sausage
- Shellfish
- Venison

Dairy

- Butter
- Cheese, processed
- Ice cream

- Yogurt

Other Foods

- Black tea
- Cocoa
- Coffee
- Ketchup
- Mustard
- Pepper
- Soft drinks
- Vinegar

Alkaline Foods To Enjoy

For a general rule, you're going to want to concentrate on consuming fruits and vegetables (with the exception of a few items). The "Go" list contains a few foods, including quinoa. You will find products asking for coconut oil and sesame oil as far as the oil goes. You will have these at the daily pharmacy. The baking recipes most frequently call for coconut flour, which these days is either accessible on daily markets or can be conveniently procured online. For more references for such products, check out the Resources portion. Here's the compilation of "Go" things to enjoy!

Alkalizing Fruits

- Apple
- Apricot
- Avocado
- Banana
- Berries
- Blackberries
- Cantaloupe
- Cherry, sour
- Coconut, fresh
- Currant
- Date, dried
- Fig, dried
- Grape
- Grapefruit
- Honeydew melon
- Lemon
- Lime
- Muskmelon
- Nectarine
- Orange
- Peach
- Pear
- Pineapple

- Raisins
- Raspberry
- Rhubarb
- Strawberry
- Tangerine
- Tomato
- Tropical fruits
- Umeboshi plum
- Watermelon

Alkalizing Proteins

- Almond
- Chestnut
- Millet
- Tempeh, fermented
- Tofu, fermented
- Whey protein powder

Alkalizing Seasonings and Spices

- Chili pepper
- Cinnamon
- Curry
- Ginger
- Herbs, all
- Miso

- Mustard
- Sea salt
- Tamari

Alkalizing Sweeteners

- Stevia

Alkalizing Vegetables

- Alfalfa
- Barley grass
- Beet greens
- Beets
- Broccoli
- Cabbage
- Carrot
- Cauliflower
- Celery
- Chard greens
- Chlorella
- Collard greens
- Cucumber
- Daikon
- Dandelion
- Dandelion root
- Dulce

- Edible flowers
- Eggplant
- Fermented vegetables
- Garlic
- Green beans
- Green peas
- Kale
- Kohlrabi
- Kombu
- Lettuce
- Maitake
- Mushroom
- Mustard greens
- Nori
- Onions
- Parsnip
- Pea
- Pepper
- Pumpkin
- Radish
- Reishi
- Rutabaga
- Sea vegetables
- Shiitake

- Spinach, green
- Spirulina
- Sprouts
- Sweet potato
- Tomato
- Wakame
- Watercress
- Wheat grass
- Wild greens

Other

- Apple cider vinegar
- Bee pollen
- Fresh fruit juice
- Green juices
- Lecithin granules
- Molasses, blackstrap
- Probiotic cultures
- Soured dairy products
- Vegetable juices
- Water, alkaline antioxidant
- Water, mineral

Tips: for Creating Alkaline Balance In Your Body

1. Eat plenty of Superfood fruits and vegetables It is the only thing you should do to better detox the health.

Put the veggies sliced in the fridge and place on your counter a big bowl of bright fruit to snack on.

Serve salad for lunch and dinner; hold a salad packed beforehand with all the greens in it except salad dressing, cucumbers and tomatoes, which you can incorporate later on.

2. Eat 80 percent of alkaline diets, and 20 percent average amount acid products.

3. Chew well your saliva is alkaline and you will produce two gallons a day!

4. Drink 2-3 liters of fresh water a day (not tap) Drinking alone will make all the difference because many people are left dehydrated with all the acidic contaminants.

Standard water is essentially acidic and neutralizing it is a slow process if your body is every acid.

For eg, one glass of coke, which is really acid, requires about 30 glasses of water to wash out. That's so many people prefer alkaline water that will immediately alkalize the body more easily and more efficiently.

5. Breathing for additional strength With sufficient fuel, bodies work faster.

That will help move the acids out of your body as well. Begin to take a deep breath into your belly.

This is best done in a yoga class. So that you can focus without interruption on your breathing, lie down on your bed and breathe deeply and comfortably into the belly.

Do it every day before you do it every day automatically.

6. Stop processed products: This is packed with extremely acid-forming toxic sweeteners, preservatives, toxic chemical compounds and food coloring.

In fact, the body has to work really hard to flush these contaminants out.

7. Seek opportunities to generate calm in your body and be seeing the birds or calming songs, meditating, wandering through nature ... do whatever induces peace inside you.

8. Live in daytime light: They require sunshine.

Go on runs, open the curtains and go to bed early enough for the sun to come up.

9. Get enough sleep: Inadequate sleep results in overworked and depressed body and mind.

10. Just because a food produces acid does not mean it is evil!

It's not about eliminating a whole food family or some food at all - it's about maintaining harmony.

Start the Alkaline Diet Now

It is always the toughest thing to get going. Starting may be intimidating, it can sound at first, because even though you feel like you're eager to get going, some very easy-to-fix errors will render following the alkaline diet even easier than it needs to be.

Here are my main Tips: for getting the alkaline diet going immediately. When you now adopt these rules you will see the results in 24 hours 'time.

Commence hydrating now!

I can't emphasize how vital this is, and how much you're going to gain from it. It is believed that we are continuously, permanently dehydrated as much as 90 per cent. It is also insane to deprive our body of oxygen. The body needs water for too many things, and mass intake is the simplest thing in the universe! Right now, just go to your tap and have a big glass of tea. You really don't feel better? Immediately-because it's not about emotionally good, don't you feel psychologically better? And Positive.

Even when you're studying it, don't put off your hydration-start consuming water now. Too many, then? Drink at least 2 liters a day, and strive for 1/2 oz of water a pound of body weight to drink.

Transition – Don't do anything at once!

The single largest explanation that people struggle to remain alkaline in my six years of teaching people on the alkaline diet is because they want to be flawless and achieve it at once. Have it not. Change: Change.

And it is up to you to change. You could:

- Select one meal and focus on only making the meal time correct for a week, and then pass on to the next one
- Pick 3 days a week to keep them alkaline
- Start incorporating a couple of different items a day, such as spinach or vegetables, etc.
- Start extracting acids one at a time, such as coffee or tea.

Get your Green!

However, I suggest bringing greens straight into your life. Perhaps the safest way is to quickly continue bringing the positive ones in and think about eventually taking the negative stuff back. My advice is to continue using a green powder including pH Miracle Greens, Regular Greens by Alkamind or Super Greens by Perfectly Safe as soon as possible. This will continue to infuse the body directly with the benefits of extremely concentrated green veggies, grasses, alkaline fruits and tons of other goodies.

It's also suggested that you start providing a salad with each meal (for now, aside from breakfast). Even though it's a little side salad, fall into the habit. There is nothing to be romantic about, just some spinach, cabbage, tomato and cucumber wrapped in lemon and olive oil. It will take 2 minutes to cook, which should render far more alkaline at mealtime. Plus, it can add at least 2 serves of 5-7 serves of veg a day to your regular need.

Core Vitamins In regards to vitamins, I can prescribe four main supplements for anyone who is on the alkaline diet and needs to become alkaline as soon as they can: 1. Green Drink: Heavily alkalising, rich with high nutrients and extremely healthy for health, green beverages are a must for me. I can almost promise that if you start getting four green drinks a day you'll start enjoying the results nearly immediately. A rich source of chlorophyll, vitamins, minerals, enzymes and other nutrients – the greens infuse the body with extremely alkaline products to cleanse, neutralize acids and give the body an immense boost of strength.

2. PH Drops: play a vital role in increasing the pH of the water you drink. It really is really essential because regular drinking water is normally acidic. So although keeping properly hydrated really is necessary, if the water is acidifying, this can be counterproductive. PH declines are extremely concentrated and produce very alkaline mineral-forming solutions. Only a few decreases would lift the pH of the water significantly.

Another advantage for pH drops like puripHy is that it has the added value of eliminating the yeasts, molds and bacteria from the water-keeping your normal drinking water very clean and alkaline!

3. Omega Oils: I firmly advise you to concentrate on the omega 3, 6, 9 and coconut oil you drink for optimal wellness, strength and wellbeing. Here's a summary of each of the key details to get you going!

* Omega 3: ALA, EPA and DHA are primary omega 3's. The human body is unable to generate omega 3 naturally, and it is necessary that we complement our diets. Omega 3 is therefore the fat we most lack of. Experts say that to work optimally we require about 20-40ml of omega 3 a day. It's impossible to achieve this from eating alone, even though we eat fatty fish and nuts every day. Particularly when many foods (including fish and meat) are produced in a way that renders them less nutritious than in the past few days

* Omega 6: LA and GLA are Omega 6's that are present in safflower, sunflower, cotton, sesame that flax. Know, however, that when oils are exposed to light, soil, or fire they are poisonous, and 99 percent of the widely used sunflower and safflower oils are worthless for health purposes. Use these natural and new on salads, pastas etc. (or all of the oils listed here) is a perfect way to improve the amount of good fats in your diet. But note – in reality, many of us eat so many omega 6 in comparison to omega 3 which can trigger problems (it is crucial to get the ratio between 3, 6 and 9).

* Omega 9: Omega 9 is predominantly OA, present in exquisite olives, nuts, avocado and macadamia oils. Again, the ratio is essential because many of us use fewer of these oils, so we don't need to weigh too much. The realistic part is that both of these oils taste good, and they can quickly be integrated into our lives.

* Short chain Coconut Oil tryglycerides (MCT): MCT is hard to get through because almost all the other oils we drink are long chain. We mention coconut oil as it is almost always raw, it is extremely immune to fire, light and air (as compared to all other oils) and it can be cooked with and always safe and it tastes fantastic!

As stated, these Essential Fatty Acids (EFAs) are considered necessary, since they are completely needed to operate by the body, and they can not be created by themselves. Eating such fats, including omega 3 and omega 6, depends on us to. Such fats are so significant that we will all ultimately perish if we did not eat all of these EFAs even if we removed the bad fats from our diets completely. Without such fats, we absolutely can not exist!

4. Alkaline salts: The alkaline salts are just too amazing. Such salts, which are centered on the four most alkaline natural salts: calcium, sodium, potassium and magnesium, are extremely alkalising and essential to life.

Note – not 100 percent 80/20

It is a major one to consider! You're not expecting an alkaline 100 per cent! You're looking for an alkaline to 20 percent acid ratio of around 80 per cent. It is a massively important thing to consider. It ensures that during your meal time you will also get a little pasta, beans, lean meats, fish etc – as long as that just occupies 20 percent of the plate due to 80 percent being filled by alkaline-forming products.

This makes it so unbelievably simple!

Chapter Two

How Acidic Wastes Cause Disease

How Acidic Wastes Causes Disease Detoxification is far more essential than proper diet for longevity. French physiologist Alexia Carrell kept fragments of chicken cardiac tissue living in a solution with the same mineral amounts present in chicken blood plasma for twenty-eight years. The cells in the tissue started dividing and died out only after he began adjusting the water, while he persisted putting the same quantity of minerals in the water. While being supplied with the required nutrients, the chicken heart cells were unable to carry out their metabolic tasks since the fluid they were put in had been contaminated with acid waste.

The human body's atmosphere can't be that quickly filtered as Carrell's chicken heart tissue test-tube world. The detoxifying organs of the body — liver, glands, digestive system, kidneys, and lungs — were not intended to neutralize toxic substances and toxins of heavy metals that have found their way through the bloodstream in recent years.

Edible oils 'hydrogenation leaves residues of aluminum and nickel behind, and food products produce fragments of such harmful heavy metals as cadmium, arsenic, mercury, and chrome. Arsenic from dental amalgams and dried tuna products, formaldehyde and arsenic in vaccination, and vehicle exhaust lead are only a handful among the multitudes among contaminants that have made a way through the bloodstream. Heavy metals migrate in the bloodstream at a higher pace when the body gets older and have bone attachment.

Lead particularly replaces calcium in the bone. So heavy metals may cause the development of bone cancer by removing the machinery in the bones that produce blood. Many products like chelators and EDTA (a mild acid used in chelation) transfer metals from the bones towards the brain where they become more harmful. "Luckily there are ways we can support the body the the arsenal of heavy metals and toxic chemicals.

A juice produced from vegetables that are rich in alkaline minerals such as celery and parsley will neutralize heavy lung metals. Lemon juice is usually an efficient detoxifier with heavy metals in the water before tea. The lemon in the water binds with positively charged metal molecules through its strong concentration of negatively charged ions, which neutralizes them. When neutralized, they are removed by the body without question.

Mineral compounds also tend to reduce heavy metals. Calcium, iron, and copper lower rates of lead; vitamin C, magnesium, and selenium extract mercury from the body; and silver, copper, and iron lower levels of cadmium.

The body also has another means to remove any of the strong acids leaching from toxins, heavy metals, and food contaminants and accumulating in the tissue. Yet they are not removed by this method. It is about keeping them out of the way of damage. If the acidity of these alien intruders reaches the mildly alkaline blood pH of the body, the body attaches them to calcium, an alkaline element, and removes them from the flowing blood as much as possible.

Acidity and Cardiovascular Disease

Acidic pollution is not necessarily made less toxic despite being securely entombed in layers of calcium. If the acidic load of the body is too growing, some acid particles linger in the blood. Through producing marks and bruises on the internal walls of arteries, they cause the initiation of cardiovascular disease. Like fat, triglycerides, magnesium, and other contaminants, these diseases are "bandaged." The greater the rates of cholesterol and triglyceride, the heavier the "bandage" and the thinner the arteries, of example

A high degree of cholesterol isn't the root source of artery hardening. Cholesterol and other thick, sticky compounds can't bind to smooth vessel walls. Just after acid particles pit and scrape the surfaces of the arterial pipe are fatty plaques allowed to adhere to them.

Of two factors, narrowed arteries are risky. Fatty plaques are more likely to become separated from the walls of the vessel and induce the development of blood clots that migrate to the brain and cause strokes across the bloodstream. These often raise blood pressure, causing heart problems and strokes more possible.

The clinical trials that effectively reduced the blood pressure in several of his patients with alkaline water suggest that the damage to arterial walls by acidic particles is the main cause of high blood pressure.5 Normalized blood pressure tests showed that the arteries had expanded and the alkaline particles in the water had dissolved the fatty plaques and acidic waste

Acidity, Autoimmune Diseases, and Protein Allergies
An unfriendly microbe is placed the foundations for autoimmune illness as the immune cells determine a certain item. The immune cells not only cause the development of histamines to "shield" the body against this "rival," but also manipulate an enzyme to create an intestinal leak. Some food molecules that the immune cells have marked as aggressive slipping into these gaps, not realizing what the immune system is up to, when they are sitting ducks for the immune cells inside the general circulation

Nevertheless, the latter get inflamed and mutate in the course of disposing of the food allergens. The immune cells target protoplasm in their own body under their current form. Evidence that it's not necessary to turn the immune system from a "Doc. Hyde "is the possibility that 63 scientifically documented autoimmune diseases, including celiac disease, lupus, rheumatoid arthritis and osteoarthritis, type 1 diabetes, and Crohn's disease, are already prevalent.

To prevent autoimmune disorder stop consuming things you already you resistant to, check yourself because you're not exactly what certain things are. Notice however that any signs, no matter how different they might appear from those triggered by food allergies, can also be related to them. Rashes, eczema, itching, nausea, vomiting, drowsiness, dizziness, arthritic discomfort and sleeplessness are the most common symptoms induced by histamines.

Acidity and cancer

Although the coronary system's wellbeing is more affected by damage caused on the heart by acid ions, the other organs of the body — liver, pancreas, kidneys, and so on — are more prone to degenerate as acidic waste accumulates in the surrounding capillaries that support it. Acid deposits thicken the blood, and the blood that is coagulated can not contain the sum of nutrition and oxygen that the kidneys require to work properly.

If we're talking to organ dysfunction, we just say the dysfunctional activity of the millions of cells that make up any organ. Among other items, these cells rely on oxygen for processing energy and amino acids for protein synthesis and for the transformation of old cells into new ones. Once such chemicals are stripped of the tissue, it then dies or adapts by being malignant to the new oxygen-deprived environment. For two factors the cancer cell can be residing in such an area. Firstly, it receives its energy from fermentation, a cycle that takes place without oxygen. Third, it constantly multiplies and collects the foods that are reserved for the regular cells of the body. The above, robbed of their sustenance, are either eaten up by fast-growing cancer cells, or avoid dividing before die.

Clearly, cancer prevention will begin with the removal of acidic waste from the body which makes normal cells cancerous. If an person is being treated for cancer, eliminating chemotherapy-generated acidic wastes may avoid a recurrence.

Acidity and Depression Acidic and Alkaline Foods
Achieving a Balance six diets are identified for people with psychiatric illnesses in his book Bio Balance. Wiley allocated certain diets similar to their acid-alkaline blood pH to the

participants of his study. There are many explanations that this diet cannot function.

Second, there is a divergence of opinion as to increasing acid producing products and growing formation alkaline. Zen Buddhists, for example, find bananas, avocados, asparagus, artichokes, and spinach to be acid-producing, whereas Western scientists claim they are alkaline since, when burnt, they leave more alkaline mineral ashes behind than acidic ones.

In addition, many acid-forming vegetables growing pH-balancing nutritionists warn us to eat less are nonetheless quite successful in reducing acidic waste. Despite their large concentration of acid-forming minerals — sulfur and phosphorus — the juice of carrots and beets successfully cleanse the toxic waste from the liver, lungs, and bladder. Cabbage extract, rich in acid-forming chlorine and arsenic, purifies the toxic acids that bind to the mucous membranes of the stomach and intestinal tract. The extremely acidic vitamin C is an ideal treatment for gum disorder and for diseases in general.

Alkaline minerals also have efficient cleaning agents. In dandelions, endive, and spinach, potassium, calcium, sodium, and magnesium decreases hyperacidity in all organs; Indeed, acid and alkaline minerals work together to cleanse the body even like a mixed solution of vinegar (acid) and soda (alkaline) bicarbonate renders an ideal cleaner for the kitchen.

Acid Alkaline Imbalance or Chronic Low-Grade Metabolic Acidosis

An important feature in naturopathic wellbeing is the acid-base balance. The equilibrium is regulated by food, consistency and quantity of liquids, respiration, suddenness and physical and psycho-emotional behavior. Of example, all living organisms continue to acidify, but it's very obvious from recent evidence that the Western diet is very acidic. The phenomenon is rising enormously in western culture, so much so that persistent acidosis is of interest to nearly all because of industrial food.

Acidification factors are mainly attributed to acidifying foods, deficiency in alkaline materials, heat, lack or abundance of physical exercise, bad water intake and insufficient respiration.

Even, in conjunction with a poor alkalizing diet (fruits, beans, nuts and seeds), too much acid-forming products (meat, sugar, starch, coffee, alcohol) produces low-level persistent acidosis. The body will use its own stocks of alkaline minerals to neutralize the extra acid. The bones contain the body's main alkali reservoir which is also found in the teeth.

Acidosis may also induce a lot of weakness, because an acidic atmosphere interferes with energy supply from body cells. Acidosis often reduces the oxygen supply available for cell operation, impacting its replication and allowing pathogenic microorganisms to expand. Acidosis frequently provides breeding ground for inflammation, and may contribute to other health issues, such as

Osteoporosis Rheumatism, gout Sciatica, herniated disk Arthritis, osteoarthritis dental caries Gum inflammation, Tooth ulcers, herpes, Fractures in the edges of the tongue, eczema, skin conditions varicose veins Colds, pneumonia, sore throat Bronchitis, sinusitis, otitis Gastric acid reflux

Understanding the conditions that support acid-base equilibrium, the collection of alkalizing and acidifying products and alkalizing food additives is an important method for combating persistent low-level acidosis.

Eventually, maintaining the body's acid-base equilibrium will restore strength and resilience.

It is important to note that it is not the stomach acid or the stomach pH that we are thinking about. We are concerned about the pH of the entirely separate substances and tissues in the body.

The pH, or "hydrogen potential," is a unit of calculation of a solution's degree of acidity or alkalinity. It is placed on a scale from 0 to 14.

A mixture of acid and alkaline substances is expressed by PH 7 or "balanced pH."

A low pH of 7 to 0 implies acidity, A Strong pH of 7 to 14 suggests alkalinity A small increase of pH leads to a significant shift in the concentration of hydrogen ions, 10 times greater from unit to unit: pH 7 = neutral pH 6 = 10 times higher acid pH 5 = 10 x 10 = 100 times more acid than neutral pH 4 = 10 x 100 = 1,000 times more acid than neutral.

When you are fit, have a good lifestyle and a safe, nutritious food, the pH in the urine will be about 7.

Between meals, it is advised to test the pH 3 times a day and the second urination in the morning, since the first urination is always acid.

Check the body's acidity or alkalinity with pH strips: Monitor the pH values and decide whether the body needs urgent treatment. By using a pH check strip, you can rapidly and conveniently evaluate the pH element in the comfort of your own home. If the urinary pH fluctuates from 6.0 and 6.5 in the morning and 6.5 and 7.0 in the evening, the body should work within a safe spectrum of conditions. If your saliva remains during the day between 6.5 and 7.5 your body functions within a safe range, an hour before a meal and two hours following a meal is the perfect time to check your pH. Check the heart rate twice a week.

Acidic Waste Causes Alcohol Addiction

How do acidic wastes from drug by-products and undigested food debris generate a taste for drug? The acid ions caused by histamines build up to acidify the blood with the continuous intake of allergy-causing products. The enhanced acidification of the alkaline blood pH elicits an adrenal response. We increase the development of the stress-promoting hormones, as the adrenals consider hyperacidity as a warning that the safety of the organism is under attack. (That's because rage and anxiety both increase blood acid levels.) However since in fact there's no risk, there's no trigger for the individual's desire to get involved in a violent action. This causes anxiety that generates a desire for anything — food, alcoholic beverages, caffeinated beverages, or cigarettes — that can relieve the strain. That disease these individuals take hold depends on where their physical weakness resides. Although an alarm response, caused by hyperacidity, initiates the decline into intoxication, the cravings for alcohol are intensified if the alcoholic beverages and the liver can not neutralize the alcohol's acid aldehyde by-product. This constant assault on the liver induces more serious hangovers — headaches, dizziness, irritability, tremor, and a loss of balance. The stronger the hangover, the more severe the drug cravings become, which is why drinking becomes worse over time.

Alcohol and the Brain

After the liver, the brain is the next most vulnerable organ to the damaging effects of chronic alcohol consumption because its energy needs are greater than those of any other organ in the body. In advanced stages of alcoholism, the brain doesn't get the glucose and oxygen needed for the production of energy. The alcoholic liver is not able to supply the brain with these raw materials, and blockages in the small blood vessels prevent them from delivering energy-generating oxygen and glucose to the brain.

Such blockages arise as they collect in the blood as the liver is no longer able to absorb toxic contaminants that allow the red blood cells to bind together. Acidic Blood pollution often creates bacteria that feed on it. The result is clumps of agglutinous material that clog the blood vessels throughout the body so that there is very little space in the blood for glucose, oxygen, and other nutrients. Without these raw materials needed to produce cellular energy and for the repair and regeneration of the cells, brain function breaks down and the neurons drown in their own metabolic waste.

There may be another factor in the brain of the alcoholic that prevents it from generating energy. The brains of hamsters, put on a diet of alcohol for experimental purposes, couldn't use glucose as a fuel. This indicates that it isn't always a lack of glucose that prevents the alcoholic brain from meeting its energy needs but the inability of the brain to use it. Besides glucose, however, there is a substance that the brain may use for food, and that's L-glutamine. The L-glutamine is transformed to glutamic acid as it reaches the blood-brain barrier. It is suspected that the brain can use glutamic acid to manufacture energy because it reduces excess ammonia, a toxic compound (from the breakdown of amino acids) that probably destroys glucose before it has a chance to enter the brain cells and be oxidized.

The healing effects of both niacin and L-glutamine, obtained by the neutralization and elimination of acid waste and alien chemicals, serve as a reminder that toxicity—which is almost overwhelmingly acidic in nature—is the fundamental cause of alcoholism. But the addiction for alcohol manifests itself only if there is an adrenal weakness that causes wild swings in blood sugar and/or an enzyme deficiency that prevents the liver from breaking down the toxic by-products of alcohol.

In many cases, however, these weaknesses cause alcohol addiction only when the diet is not compatible with the metabolism. An inappropriate or junk-food diet triggers the actions of adrenal hormones that disrupt the concentration and normal distribution of sugar—one of the most important factors in metabolic function. The first step, then, in a program designed to overcome alcoholism is for the individual to take the niacin self-test to find out whether to go on the meat eater's or grain eater's diet.

Cirrhosis of the Liver

Not only does putting the body on emergency alert (adrenal overstimulation) create anxiety and tension that drives some people to alcoholism, but it also starts a cycle of reactions that ultimately destroy the liver. The liver, responding to the alert from the adrenals to raise blood sugar levels, takes an excessive amount of glucose out of storage and releases it into the bloodstream.

Because there is really no need for this sudden rise in blood sugar, an increase in insulin produced by the beta cells in the pancreas drastically lowers blood sugar levels, causing hypoglycemia (low blood sugar). Low blood sugar means sluggish energy production, which interferes with liver function. It can also cause fatigue and depression, symptoms that, like anxiety, increase the craving for alcohol. As long as the individual continues drinking and acid levels in the blood remain high, the adrenals will direct the liver to raise blood sugar excessively and insulin will respond by reducing it precipitously.

Eventually the liver can't comply with the adrenal hormones' request for more glucose because it no longer has any. (The liver keeps glucose in the nature of glycogen.) One reason for this is that the drinker, preferring alcohol to food, doesn't supply the liver with the carbohydrates, protein, and fat it needs to make glucose. Another is the presence of fat, which should pass out of the liver into general circulation but can't because of alcohol's destruction of the B vitamin choline. (The absence of choline prevents fat from being converted by the liver into phospholipids, which can pass through phospholipid molecules in the cellular membrane of the cells in the liver into the bloodstream.) So fat molecules, remaining in the liver and needing a place to park themselves, fill up the spaces in the liver that are designed to store glucose. Fatty deposits also replace liver cells that have been destroyed by the alcoholic by-product, acid aldehyde. As if that weren't enough, metabolic wastes and acid aldehyde inflame the liver by destroying oxygen. Inflamed tissue develops scars, just like a wound or incision does.

But scar tissue on the surface of the skin is harmless, whereas scar tissue in the liver destroys its ability to function by impeding circulation. An almost nonexistent blood supply turns the liver tissue into hard fibers, a sign that the liver has developed cirrhosis, a disease that, without early nutritional intervention, is fatal.

Can the recovered alcoholic heal the brain damage caused by the brain's inability to generate energy? Studies conducted by researchers at the Massachusetts General Hospital and Boston

University using MRI images reveal that long-term abstinence from alcohol does bring some cognitive recovery.

Nevertheless, the most vulnerable portion of the brain rarely regains. It is the amygdala limbic network, where anxiety and anger start, and the hippocampus, where long-term memories are processed. The capacity of the amygdala to provide the requisite neurons that enable us to understand what facial gestures signify is forever impaired, including in the long-term abstinent alcoholics. But giving up drinking helps in the gradual regeneration of the prefrontal cortex, the most newly formed portion of the brain.

Acidic Waste and Cardiovascular Problems

What caused Sam's arteries to harden after they had been cleared of cholesterol, calcium, and various other kinds of debris? A question more to the point is, why did they harden in the first place? As usual, scientific researchers have looked in the wrong direction. Ignoring the true cause of the calcified plaques lining the arteries—injuries inflicted on the arteries by sharp crystals of acidic waste—they have come up with a culprit called cytomegalovirus that invades the body and implants itself inside the walls of the arteries.

Several studies support the connection between the presence of this virus and the regrowth of plaque. In one study of seventy-five patients who had had an angioplasty, fatty plaque recurred in 75 percent of those patients who were infected with the cytomegalovirus, while only 8 percent who were not infected had a recurrence of plaque. Another research indicates that those with no signs of heart failure who were taking tetracycline were 30 percent less likely to experience a heart attack than people who did not take antibiotics.

Acidic Waste Virus and Bacteria Induce Arterial Hardening Which may seem to be strong proof that the cytomegalovirus is the source of artery hardening. Nevertheless, the truth is that the presence of this virus in the bloodstream is clarified by the acidic waste that circulates in the blood (from undigested food debris). Viruses and bacteria feed on acidic waste, and reproduce. In this respect, it is instructive to note the bitter conclusion that the renowned German pathologist Rudolf Virchow (1821–1902) came to work on the basis of the conviction that germs were the source of disease after investing a lifetime: "If I could live my life again, I would dedicate it to showing that germs try their natural habitat — diseased tissues. Mosquitoes, for example, try the stagnant water but do not allow the pool to stagnate.

Studies demonstrate that in the short term, antibiotics, vaccines, and strong anti-inflammatory drugs eliminate megalovirus infections, preventing the regrowth of plaque after an angioplasty. But no studies have been made on the long-term effectiveness of these treatments. It seems unlikely that the health of the arteries can be maintained indefinitely even with the use of antibiotics to kill off the cytomegalovirus, when the condition that caused the original inflammation is not addressed—the acid waste circulating in the arterial blood that damages the arteries and provides nourishment for the cytomegalovirus.

In nature, bacteria and viruses live off the acidic tissue of dead organisms—they are nature's primary decomposers. The acid waste from undigested food circulating in the blood provides germs in the blood with the same kind of acidic brew that the dead bodies of wild animals and plants provide the bacteria in nature.

Acidic waste particles make scratches and tears on the inside walls of the blood vessels. The injured cells die off and turn into acidic waste, adding to its accumulation in the blood. The larger the quantities of acidic waste the greater the food supply for germs; they multiply correspondingly. This forces the immune system to defend the walls of the arteries by triggering the growth of tumors to encapsulate germ colonies, causing further damage to the arterial walls.

The immune system also patches the injuries in the lining of the vessels with calcified plaques to prevent life-threatening leaks, and it reacts to arterial degeneration the same way it does to bodily injury from accidents—by triggering the flow of blood to the area that inflames the walls of the arteries. Such steps avoid mortality from inevitable yet create the stage for a heart attack. All that needs to do is for the creation of a blood clot, preventing blood supply to the neck. This will happen as a calcified plaque falls out at the surface of the vessel.

Nausea, a sense of suffocation, dizziness and fainting spells, tightness in the throat, or discomfort in the heart area or left arm followed by sensations of fear are the most frequent signs of a heart attack. However, if a chest pain happens concurrently with cold hands and feet, and air becomes shallow, it is typically a symptom of indigestion.

Chapter Three

Achieving Ph Balance To Treat Specific Ailments

DIGESTIVE AILMENTS

Acid waste, under ideal conditions, is nothing more than the by product of all the physical and chemical processes that go on in the body. Such acid waste is easily neutralized and removed by way of sweat, urine, and stool. But when there is—in addition to this naturally occurring acid waste in the body—acidic waste from the breakdown of undigested food, the body can't dispose of all of it. In this situation, acid waste causes health problems. The first to show up is usually acid indigestion, most particularly, acid reflux.

Acid Reflux

Acid reflux, accompanied by a pain in the throat and arms, happens as the acid discharge from undigested food passes through the esophagus (throat) from the stomach. Unlike the lungs, there's no dense mucous coating on the esophagus to shield it from the contaminants 'hard acid crystals. If acid reflux is persistent it allows the esophageal tissues to swell and red. This may contribute to esophagus deterioration, and consequently cancer.

High rates of stomach acid waste can cause gastric problems such as spastic stomach, duodenal ulcers and inflammation of the intestines. (The duodenum, the uppermost portion of the small intestine, is connected to the bottom of the stomach.) Signs of acid indigestion may be a life-saver, since they indicate the acidic waste in the digestive tract exceeds harmful amounts and thus therefore accumulates in certain areas of the body.

Sooner or later excessive acid waste gives rise to degenerative disease. Many individuals, however, develop debilitating illness without having any symptoms of acid indigestion; with no gastric symptoms, they don't see the link between poor digestion and diseases in the organ systems outside the digestive tract.

For those with acid reflux, gastritis (stomach inflammation), diarrhea, bloating, gallstones and ulcers, where eating is an apparent culprit, find it impossible to understand that products that induce intestinal symptoms will often destroy organs that are not part of the digestive system. However, any malaise and discomfort in the body that is not the consequence of physical damage or hereditary predisposition is caused by unhealthy and/or nutrient-deficient nutritional acidic waste materials.

Unfortunately for their patients, conventional physicians treat disease effects as indicators of sickness rather than as responses to metabolically unhealthy foods. Mary's been a survivor of the strategy. Six years earlier, on her way home from a wedding, her pulse started to pound, her hands trembled and she had a seizure minutes later. Since scans tested inaccurate, the doctor believed that she was getting the flu.

But instead of getting over the "flu," she developed shivering fits, felt tremendous pressure in her head, and could hardly hold herself up.

After she had seven seizures in one week, the doctor conducted more extensive tests. An EEG (electroencephalogram), performed while she slept, showed that her brain waves were off the charts: 1:2 is normal; hers had slowed to 1:600. A blood workup revealed that she had an adrenal insufficiency and her antibodies were so elevated that they were a strong indication of an autoimmune disorder. The doctor suspected lupus.

Mary was already taking antiseizure medication and was now told that she should take prednisone, a steroid hormone, and undergo cytotoxin chemotherapy. She decided that these drugs were the proverbial straws that would break the camel's back, in this case hers, so she took matters into her own hands and went to a naturopathic physician. The first thing that the naturopath did was to test for allergies.

The tests indicated that Mary was allergic to wheat, sugar, dairy, caffeine, alcohol, bananas, and potatoes. She went on an allergy-free diet, and in a few days her symptoms disappeared. She regained her sense of well-being, alertness, and ability to concentrate two to three weeks later. The nightmare was over.

Thinking back on her illness, what frightens her most is the fact that as sick as she was, she had no symptoms of indigestion from her food allergies and therefore no clue as to why she was so ill. Mary's experience shows that the role of diet in initiating an illness should be the first consideration even when there are no symptoms of indigestion.

A mixture of acidic particles (positively charged protons) and alkaline particles (negative charged electrons) constitute the basic framework of the elements — primarily carbon, nitrogen, oxygen, and hydrogen — from which all the tissues in the body are created. (Neutrons in the nucleus of atoms have no charge.) If a substance contains more electrons than protons, it is charged negatively (hydroxyl ions, OH-), and if it contains more protons than electrons, it is charged positively (hydrogen ions, H+). This made me realize the full implications of having acid indigestion. If it caused an imbalance in the acid-alkaline ratios of the blood and other fluids in the body, any or all of my organ systems could malfunction and deteriorate.

The Real Cause of Acid Reflux

Doctors have tried to cure acid reflux through surgery, repairing the valve between the stomach and esophagus to keep it from opening up and letting stomach acids pour into the esophagus. In view of the fact that the results of this operation have been disappointing, there has to be another explanation for acid reflux. The most likely one is that acidic waste gas molecules in the stomach open the valve that closes off the stomach from the esophagus by causing it to go into a spasm. (This valve should remain closed except when we eat.) Acidic waste flows through this opening, inflaming the esophagus. Chronic inflammation wears away the esophageal tissues.

Efficient digestion depends on the alternating actions of acid and alkaline digestive juices. The alkaline enzyme ptyalin in the mouth breaks down starch; hydrochloric acid and acidic gastric juices, such as pepsin, break up protein in the stomach; in the small intestine alkaline pancreatic enzymes complete the digestion of protein, and alkaline bile emulsifies fats and oils. Acid reflux can disrupt this acid-alkaline sequence by changing the pH factor in the stomach and small intestine.

How this happens is revealed by the typical contents of the stomach that heartburn sufferers sometimes throw up in an effort to get rid of the burning sensation in the throat and chest. After a highly acidic liquid is brought up, alkaline-forming bile often follows, indicating that the bile has flowed from the small intestine into the stomach, where it doesn't belong. This occurs when the pyloric valve between the stomach and small intestine opens, most likely because the acid waste causes the muscles in the valve to relax. The alkaline-forming bile in the stomach alkalinizes the acidic gastric juices, thus interfering with the stomach's breakdown of protein. As a result not only does the undigested protein turn into acid waste, but the alternating acid-alkaline balance in the digestive tract is disrupted.

Gelatin Supplies Mucilage

Powdered okra and beet juice as effective hydrophilic colloids (sticky substances that have an affinity for water) but believed the most practical and effective musilagenous substance was gelatin taken with each meal, either sprinkled on food or added to liquid. For an individual with alcoholic-related gastritis, gelatin with its enormous mucilage content is often the only remedy that will counteract the corrosive effect of alcohol on the lining of the stomach and small intestine.

Gelatin also has great nutritive value, an additional benefit for alcoholics who have lost interest in food. Edgar Cayce in one of his readings stated that gelatin aids in the absorption of vitamins and minerals. Because the calcium in gelatin (45 percent of gelatin consists of calcium) is derived from chicken bones, it's the most easily assimilated form of that mineral.

Ulcers

My mother was fed cow's milk as a baby and continued to drink it until, at the age of five, the chronic rash on her face and arms was diagnosed as an allergic reaction to milk. I suspect that the gallbladder attacks she began having in her early thirties were caused by the same chemical and/or immune system imbalance that had caused her allergy to milk as a child.

She relieved her painful gallbladder attacks, brought on by gallstones, with a hot water bottle, and the nausea that accompanied these attacks with an alkaline concoction made up of peppermint, spirits of ammonia, and sodium bicarbonate in water. A surgeon, a friend of the family, talked her into having her gallbladder removed by assuring her that, because the gallbladder's only function was storing bile, it was expendable.

(In fact, when the gallbladder is removed, the liver interprets this act as a sign that bile is no longer needed to digest fats, so it curtails its production of bile.) After removing the gallbladder, the surgeon did some exploratory surgery and discovered, much to his horror, that every inch of the lining of her stomach and duodenum (the upper part of the small intestine) was covered with ulcers. He told my mother after the operation that he regretted having taken out her gallbladder—despite the pain her gallbladder, left intact, would continue to give her—because the diet for ulcers (at the time) emphasized milk, butter, and cream. These dairy products can be digested only with the help of the large quantity of bile that can be stored in the gallbladder, so without her gallbladder my mother wouldn't have enough bile to break down the fat in butter and cream. And without this fat her ulcers wouldn't heal—or so the medical profession thought at the time. The result was that her gallbladder attacks worsened and her ulcers became seemingly permanent fixtures in her stomach and duodenum.

The Healing Quality of Raw Cabbage Juice

When my mother was in her late eighties, she finally agreed to try a natural cure for her ulcers and gallbladder attacks—raw cabbage juice. Reluctantly, she began drinking two pints of it a day, sometimes adding carrots. In only two weeks she began having fewer stomach upsets. Two months later she stopped having them altogether.

The effectiveness of raw cabbage in healing ulcers—as well as eliminating gallstones—proves that foods that contain more acid-forming minerals than alkaline ones, despite the claims otherwise, can heal the body. Raw cabbage cleans out the acid waste in the stomach, allowing ulcers to heal and the mucous membrane lining in the stomach to rebuild itself. The beneficial action of a food like cabbage on acid indigestion—with its acid-forming minerals, chlorine, phosphorous, and sulfur notwithstanding—is evidence that foods high in acidic minerals are not the cause of degenerative disease; on the contrary, they have great curative value.

The Preventive Role of Whole Grains

Many studies show that whole grains are an effective remedy for an ulcerated stomach. Where unrefined wheat is the dietary staple, for example, in northern India and China and parts of Africa, ulcers are rare. On the other hand, in Japan, where white rice has replaced the traditional brown rice as a dietary staple, peptic ulcers, once almost unheard of, have become common.

No one knows just what fiber does to heal ulcers. One theory is that it reduces gastric enzymes, which the medical establishment claims is the cause of acid reflux and ulcers. If this were the case, eating fiber-rich food would worsen ulcers, for it takes a lot of gastric enzymes to break down the fiber in grain.

The theory that fiber toughens the stomach lining has more merit, since the rough texture of fiber acts as a broom, sweeping away the irritating acidic debris lodged in the lining of the stomach. However the fact that ulcers have skyrocketed everywhere in the world since 1900—along with the rise in coronary heart disease—when the removal of the husk covering the grain became widespread, suggests that some of the benefits of fiber come from the nutrients it harbors, particularly vitamins E and B, in addition to the fact that it moves waste matter along the intestinal tract.

Because meat eaters (parasympathetic dominant) don't digest grains well, they have to satisfy most of their fiber requirements with raw fruits and vegetables, which don't have the quantity of B and E vitamins that grains have. This makes vitamin E and a multiple B supplement—preferably in the form of whole-food complexes—a necessity for those with a meat-eating metabolism who suffer from acid indigestion and ulcers.

The Mucilage in Bananas, Plantains, and Cabbage Juice

Bananas and plantains—especially green plantains—and raw cabbage juice heal ulcers by thickening the mucous lining of the stomach. Dr. Ralph Best, a British pharmacist at the University of Aston in Birmingham, observed a thickening of the stomach wall in autopsies of animals fed banana powder. Dr. Garnett Cheney, a researcher at Stanford University, wrote in the Journal of the American Dietetic Association in 1950 of his treatment of twenty-six ulcer patients with cabbage juice, twenty-four of whom made a complete recovery in three to four weeks.

Of the nineteen patients in the group treated with conventional medicines, only six recovered. Many independent investigations confirmed the research and that stomach ulcers disappeared in 85 percent of the 500 subjects in these studies.

Vermel believes that vitamin U, about which nothing is known, supplies a nutrient needed for the formation of mucus. I would say, rather, that the factor in bananas and cabbage that rebuilds the stomach's mucous lining is hyaluronic acid, the substance in mucilage that gives it its slippery and gluelike texture.

Colitis, Ileitis, and Other Inflammatory Intestinal Disorders

Bess, age sixty-six, had had colitis (inflammation of the colon) and ileitis (inflammation of the section of the small intestine that joins the colon) since her midtwenties. Like many individuals with an inflammatory intestinal condition, she had mental problems. It was an attribute she had inherited; many members of her family suffered from depression, several had committed suicide, and three of her grandparents had died of Alzheimer's disease.

Bess's anxiety led to feelings of depression so severe that they clouded over the sunny disposition she had had as a child. She came to hate herself, not just who she was but the way she looked. For twenty years she had avoided looking at herself in the mirror. The little self-esteem she possessed went into her nails, which she kept beautifully manicured. Despite all her insecurities, she charmed everyone she met and was extremely well informed on almost any topic that came up in a conversation.

Bess had been something of a child prodigy. She learned to read at the age of eighteen months and was reading a newspaper at the age of two. She has a talent similar to those of idiot savants. Without looking, she can write at the same time with both hands, her left hand writing from left to right and her right hand from right to left until her hands meet.

The most recent of Bess's colitis and ileitis attacks had occurred when she removed books from the bookshelves in her living room so they could be painted. Looking at the empty bookshelves triggered painful cramps, bloating, and diarrhea. After the shelves had been painted and the books replaced, she had an even worse attack of cramps and diarrhea. Bess had had so many bouts of diarrhea over the years that she had developed ulcerated colitis. Her inflammatory bowel disorders were synchronized with her attacks of anxiety.

Not all individuals with inflammatory intestinal problems experience the same severe stress levels as Bess, but it's hard to find anyone with this disorder who doesn't insist that it is triggered by anxiety. The stress might be the result of a major upheaval such as being fired from a job or the death of a close relative, but more likely it arises from taking on a responsibility that isn't part of the daily routine: redoing a kitchen, planning a wedding, job hunting, making preparations for a trip, working overtime, and so on.

Appendectomy

There are other causes of intestinal inflammation besides mental stress. One is the removal of the appendix. This operation, from 1900 to around 1950, was almost as common as tonsillectomy. The justification for its removal was that it was a vestigial (useless) organ. That in fact the appendix has a vital function in the body is suggested by several studies that have correlated appendectomies with an increase in cancer.

A study of 1,165 patients at the Medical College in Toledo, Ohio, conducted showed that 67 percent of the patients who had developed cancer before the age of fifty had had their appendix removed; according to his studies, out of hundreds of cancer patients, 84 percent had had their appendixes removed whereas only 25 percent of the noncancer patients were missing their appendixes.

These studies make a strong case that the appendix, like the tonsils and adenoids, is part of the immune system and as such produces antibodies that not only destroy cancer-causing viruses but also engulf and dispose of the toxins and bacteria that inflame the bowels. The appendix's location at the bottom of the ascending colon clearly indicates that its purpose is to protect the small intestine from the toxic waste in the ascending colon.

According to Michael Crichton, M.D., in his book Five Patients, appendix operations started with the pathologist Reginald H. Fitz's assertion that inflammation, pus, and pain in the lower right abdomen was caused by an infection in the appendix.

This hypothesis, Crichton writes, created a new disease. Although many physicians resisted the idea of removing the appendix, eventually the surgeons won out. The final victory for the appendix removal proponents was achieved in 1902 when England's King Edward VII had an appendectomy. Shortly afterward, the operation came into vogue. Physicians were not then aware, as most still aren't today, that inflammation from toxic acidic waste is the initial cause of appendicitis. (In China today hospitals typically offer patients with appendicitis two choices: an appendectomy or a program of herbs and diet to detoxify the appendix, thus avoiding the necessity for an operation.)

Other Causes of Inflammatory Intestinal Disorders

Doctors no longer remove the appendix as a matter of course, but this hasn't decreased inflammatory bowel disease, because new medical interventions have come into use that are damaging to the intestinal tract. Irritable bowel syndrome, Crohn's disease, and colitis became commonplace when antibiotics came into widespread use more than fifty years ago. Bacteria that survive antibiotic treatment develop a resistance to it, possibly by producing a virulent toxin that destroys the antibiotics—and also damages the intestinal walls.

The measles vaccination has also increased bowel disease. A British study of 3,545 individuals who received measles vaccinations showed that there was a threefold increase in Crohn's disease and a two-and-a-half-fold increase in ulcerative colitis as compared to a control group.The formaldehyde, mercury, and diseased animal tissue in vaccines all contribute to the breakdown of intestinal tissues.

The result of a Swedish study shows a relationship between junk food and an increase in intestinal disorders that is hardly surprising.According to the study, those who eat fast foods at least twice a week are 3.4 times more likely to develop Crohn's disease and 3.9 times more likely to develop ulcerative colitis. Junk food debris, like antibiotics, vaccines, and mental stress, produces acidic waste that triggers the flow of adrenal hormones. These hormones divert the flow of blood from the digestive tract to the cardiovascular system, the first step in the march toward inflammatory bowel disease.

Curing Inflammatory Intestinal Disorders
Bowel disorders can be relieved by reducing stress. When the calming effect is achieved, the two halves of the autonomic nervous system—the sympathetic and parasympathetic nerves—become better balanced. This balance brings on a more even distribution of the blood and lymph fluids, so that all the organ systems receive their fair share of nutrients and oxygen. This in turn improves digestion and the transit of food and waste through the digestive tract, which gives the intestines a chance to heal.

Bess healed her colitis and ileitis by relieving her anxiety and depression. She took a supplement called SAM-e. (SAM-e is activated methionine.) SAM-e increases the production of the neurotransmitters that have a calming effect and lower stress hormone levels—L-dopa, dopamine, and phosphatidylcholine. Bess also took Aangamik, which relieves depression by oxygenating the brain cells. After she had been on this regimen for several months, she no longer felt anxious over the least deviation in her daily routine, and her feelings of depression lifted. She was the first member of her family to have conquered a mental disorder. Her calmness indicated that her stress-promoting hormone levels had dropped. The resulting increase in blood flow to the intestines normalized her intestinal function.

A major cause of intestinal disorders is bad diet, which is most likely a contributing factor in cases where mental stress is the primary cause. Anyone with a bowel disorder should try to reduce intestinal inflammation by avoiding foods that produce an allergic reaction and by eating only organically grown foods based on their metabolic type. Martha's intestinal function got better when she made some changes in her diet. She tested herself for food allergies and found that she was lactose intolerant, the most common allergy in people with intestinal inflammation.

(In a study of 77 patients with irritable bowel syndrome conducted by Italian physicians, 74 percent were found to be allergic to milk. They were put on a milk-free diet for three weeks, and their condition in all cases improved.) Martha's attacks of diarrhea became less frequent but didn't go away entirely, so she took three tablespoons of bran three times a day to strengthen the intestinal walls. Eating bran on a regular basis speeds up the transit time of stool by increasing peristaltic movement.

In Martha's case, however, it acted as an irritant, causing her intestines to become more inflamed. Discouraged, she went to her family doctor for treatment. He told her that raw garlic was effective for all forms of inflammatory bowel disease but asked her to keep it confidential—what if it got around that he had recommended a folk remedy! It always worked, he said. The patient had to eat as many raw cloves of garlic as he or she could stand, fixed in a variety of different ways to make it more palatable. Martha tried the garlic remedy, and it worked just as her doctor said it would.

John started having digestive problems when he was twenty. By the time he was thirty-five he had developed Crohn's disease, an extremely severe inflammatory bowel disorder. He tried to avoid foods that gave him indigestion, but his job took him all over the world, and his digestive tract couldn't adjust to foods that differed from one country to the next. His intestines became so inflamed that the doctor prescribed prednisone, a steroid hormone. When that didn't work, he had three feet of his intestines and his ileocaecal valve removed. Fearing that if his inflamed bowel condition continued to worsen he would end up with no intestines at all, John began investigating alternative remedies. I suggested castor oil, the best remedy for a sluggish gut and one that has been used for many ailments since biblical times. The oil is extracted from the castor bean, which grows on a tree called the Palma Christi. According to Edgar Cayce, castor oil activates peristalsis in the colon by triggering a chemical action in which water splits oil into glycerol and the fatty acid ricinoleic acid.

John placed a castor oil pack on his lower abdomen for one hour every day for one week and took one tablespoon of the oil every morning before breakfast. In a week his stools, which had been either too loose or too hard, assumed a normal consistency. His abdominal cramps and pain, however, hadn't gone away because his intestines were still inflamed, a sign that his bowel was still hyperacidic. To increase the alkalinity of his intestines, John slept on a far infrared pad (see Resources). He also drank alkaline water. A month later he broke out in a rash and had open, running sores all over his abdomen. The acidic waste in his gut had been dissolved and excreted through the skin. With this removal, the pain and inflammation in John's intestinal tract vanished.

As the personal stories in this chapter reveal, the way to cure digestive tract problems is to neutralize the acid wastes in the body. While this can be done with alkaline-based products such as the infrared mat and alkaline water, clearly the most effective treatment is an allergy-free diet that takes into consideration an individual's metabolic type—meat eater, grain eater, or the balanced metabolism.

Gallbladder Problems

It is ironic that a cholesterol-rich saturated fat diet helps prevent gallstones when bile crystallizes into gallstones only when the gallbladder becomes supersaturated with cholesterol. Two siblings, John and Margaret, are examples of what happens when cholesterol is excluded from the diet. Their mother gave them plenty of vegetables, salads, and fruit, but being excessively cholesterol conscious, she served only lean meat and no butter. Margaret's and John's only source of fatty acids was olive oil in the salads they had every night with their dinner. Both suffered from constipation.

When John graduated from college and moved to his own apartment, he ate out every night at fast-food restaurants where he invariably ordered a cheeseburger and French fries. Nevertheless, from the day he left home his constipation vanished. John was now eating saturated fats, and this change in diet, despite its nutritional deficiencies and chemical additives, had solved his elimination problem. His younger sister, Margaret, however, continued to have the problem after she moved away from home. Like her mother, she avoided butter and trimmed the fat off meat. She also took birth control pills.

Five years later she stopped taking them long enough to become pregnant. About a year after she had given birth to a son, she went back on birth control pills. One night she woke up in agony. Pain from a spot under her right rib cage, where the gallbladder is located, radiated into her chest and down her left arm. Afraid that she was having a heart attack, her husband rushed her to the hospital where an MRI revealed gallstones. One of them, half an inch in diameter, was blocking her gallbladder duct. The bile, trapped in the gallbladder by the obstruction, had been diverted into the bloodstream, giving her skin and the whites of her eyes a yellowish tint. Because the gallbladder was badly inflamed, the doctors removed it.

Margaret met three of the criteria that have been linked to gallstones. She had been on a low-cholesterol diet for years, had been constipated for the same period of time, and had been taking birth control pills. A low-cholesterol diet, by causing constipation, can pave the way for gallstones. Cholesterol is one of the raw materials out of which bile salts are made. Bile salts stimulate peristalsis—the alternate contraction and relaxation of the muscles in the intestinal tract that helps overcome elimination problems. Thus a diet low in cholesterol can result in a deficiency of bile salts with the consequent slowing up of the movement of the muscles in the colon, making elimination of stool more difficult.

Constipation increases the likelihood of gallstones by causing the waste matter in the colon to putrefy and give off toxins. If these toxins can't be detoxified by the liver or kidneys, the liver incorporates them in bile. The bile is released into the gallbladder. There, it bonds with cholesterol and hardens into stone. A case control study by F. Pixley, originally published in Gut, titled "Dietary Factors in the Etiology of Gallstones," showed a relationship between stone formation and supersaturated quantities of cholesterol in the bladder.

Gallstones can also form when the liver and kidneys are too congested to process the fatty acids altered by excessive blood levels of estrogen.

Allergy-causing foods are also a factor in gallbladder attacks and the formation of gallstones. A study carried out back in the 1960s provides evidence for this claim. The 69 patients in his study, all of whom suffered from recurrent gallbladder attacks, were put on an elimination diet to determine their food allergies. Those of the 69 patients who avoided the foods they were allergic to had no more attacks. The primary offending foods were eggs (92.8 percent), pork (63.8 percent), onions (52.2 percent), chicken and turkey (34.8 percent), milk (24.6 percent), coffee (21.7 percent), and oranges (18.8 percent).

The Cholesterol Issue

Why the role of "bad guy" was in coronary heart disease assigned to cholesterol—that waxy, gray-yellow substance in our bodies that is vital to the growth of tissue, development of the brain, and manufacture of hormones? The answer lies in the mind-set of the medical establishment, which holds that when a medical problem arises, a "bad guy" is responsible: a virus, bacteria, or some substance researchers label harmful, which the body itself manufactures—such as cholesterol.

Medical researchers have ignored studies conducted by Rudolf Virchow in the nineteenth century. He discovered that degeneration of the blood vessels started before cholesterol plaques appeared in the lesions. The late Dr. G. E. Barnes reaffirmed Virchow's conclusions. He examined fifty thousand autopsies of people who died in Europe during World War II when saturated fats like meat and butter were scarce.

These autopsies showed advanced hardening of the arteries in spite of the low-cholesterol diet in individuals who had died too young to have heart attacks. Legions of statistics show similar results, among them the fourteen-year Framingham, Massachusetts, study, which found that one-half of the individuals in the study who died of heart attacks had normal cholesterol levels.4 This indicates that there is no definitive link between moderately high cholesterol and cardiovascular disease.

Heart Disease and Hormonal Imbalance

There is a relationship between heart disease and hormonal imbalance that is worth noting. Excessive acid waste in the blood from anxiety or poor diet triggers the rise of the stress-promoting hormones estrogen and cortisol. At unacceptably high levels, these hormones trigger heart disease. Excess estrogen does so by destroying oxygen, which inflames the arteries and veins. Estrogen has also been found to expand the walls of the veins carrying blood back to the heart, postponing the return of the blood to the heart and causing the heartbeat to slow.

Raw Foods Prevent Excessive Weight Gain

We should emulate, to the extent possible, the raw food–eating habits of preindustrial cultures, because for nearly all of the three hundred thousand years of protohuman's existence, everything was eaten raw. It was only with the Wurm Glacial period sixty-five thousand years ago that humans began cooking with fire, thus destroying the enzymes in foods that prevent obesity. Enzymes keep weight down, because, like workers at a construction site who use just enough bricks and mortar to put a building together, they convert the food we eat into the exact quantity of raw materials needed for maintaining and rebuilding the body. The rest is eliminated.

However, in the case of enzyme-free cooked food, there is nothing to prevent too many nutrients from being absorbed into the body's cells. What the body doesn't need is stored in fat cells located in loose connective (adipose) tissue. Cooked food also causes weight gain because, taking longer to digest, it leaves food particles behind. Leftover food turns into acidic waste, some of which is stored in the body as fat.

Unlike raw food, cooked food stimulates the endocrine glands, causing them to secrete excessive levels of hormones.This increases body weight because hormones regulate body functions. They switch body functions on and off according to the body's needs. An excessive level of hormones turns the production centers in the cells on too often, causing the overproduction of nutrients. Excess nutrients are stored in fat molecules under the skin. A study in which the effects on weight gain between canned and raw food are compared, the study concluded that canned food, which must be cooked at a high temperature, caused more weight gain than the same food left raw.

Monosodium glutamate (MSG), which is added to many bottled and canned foods as well as poultry and fast foods, is also linked to weight gain. A review of the article "Diabetes Danger in a Taste of Chinese" states that scientists have discovered that MSG affects insulin secretion.

Since MSG is known to excite the endocrine glands, it is safe to conclude that the beta cells in the pancreas that produce insulin,

when exposed to MSG, become whipped up and overproduce it.
Excessive levels of insulin lower blood sugar excessively. The
resulting low blood sugar, referred to as hypoglycemia, is
associated with obesity, probably because the excess glucose
that is removed from the blood is converted to fat. Elevated
insulin is not only associated with obesity but also with the
recurrence of breast cancer. It can be lowered by taking
pantothenic acid, a B vitamin. (Specific suggestions are given at
the end of this chapter.)

MSG is not the only artificial chemical that promotes obesity.
Any foods that are altered by chemical additives confuse the
appestat mechanism. This is the part of the brain that signals us
to eat when our stomachs are empty and our body tissues need
nourishment by creating hunger pangs. It tells us to stop when
our stomachs are full and nutrient requirements are met, by
creating a feeling of satiety. Chemicalized foods tend to
stimulate hunger, even when the body does not need nutrients.
Another factor contributing to obesity is eating food deficient in
such alkaline minerals as calcium, magnesium, and potassium.
(This includes most processed foods.) Alkaline minerals are
needed to neutralize the acidic waste that is the by-product of
even the most nutritious foods. When the supply of alkaline
minerals is low, acidic wastes don't get neutralized.

While some of the fatty acids in the waste are stored as body fat,
other fatty acids are converted to cholesterol and lactic acid.

This increases the acid levels in the blood and lymph fluids, which makes the body more vulnerable to weight gain because as blood, loaded with acidic waste, circulates, it clogs organ systems. This slows down metabolism so that correspondingly less food (fuel) is burned up.

Excessive weight gain is also caused by the consumption of refined grains. Even before our digestive enzyme glands had a chance to adjust to the kind and quantity of enzymes needed to break down the grains that had been introduced into the diet only around seven thousand years ago, manufacturers (in the early 1900s) started tampering with them by removing the husks.

The health benefits of whole grains are not just in the nutritional content. They take longer to digest than refined grains. The advantage of slow digestion is that blood sugar levels don't rise excessively. Refined grains, on the other hand, are broken down so quickly they leave behind excessive levels of glucose in the blood. This is another case where high blood sugar levels are converted by insulin to fat.

Excessive glucose in the liver is converted to fat just as it is in the blood. A fatty liver is more dangerous to health than layers of fat under the skin because the fat globules in the liver prevent it from detoxifying digested food plus performing its myriad other functions.

Chapter Four

Foods That Suppress Thyroid Function

There are also substances in certain foods that suppress thyroid function. These foods should be avoided if you have an underactive thyroid: beans (all beans except string beans); peanuts; polyunsaturated oils; undercooked broccoli, cauliflower, and cabbage; muscle meat; and beta-carotene. Goiter (enlarged thyroid) ceased to be a major health problem when iodine was added to salt, but more recently, with the use of iodide as an emulsifier in bread dough, yogurt, and pudding to make a smooth consistency, the public is getting an overload of iodine. This can interfere with the thyroid's production of thyroxin to the same extent as too little iodine and is probably one of the causes of the current epidemic of hypothyroidism. Foods that promote thyroid function are animal hearts, butter, vitamin A instead of beta-carotene, skin for its gelatin content (unless you are sensitive to MSG [monosodium glutamate]), and eggs.

Avoid Processed Foods and Water Pollutants

Thyroid function is also inhibited by the heavy metal residues found in processed foods and in food additives. Estrogen, a stress hormone, can increase the heavy metal levels in our bodies because it stimulates the absorption of iron. Excess iron depletes oxygen needed for respiration (energy production).

Avoiding processed foods that are contaminated with heavy metals improves thyroid function and lowers excess estrogen levels. This in turn prevents surplus iron from being stored in the body, which in older people becomes a problem, as an aging body absorbs heavy metals more readily than a young one.

Low thyroxin levels in the blood, which inhibit thyroid function, are also caused by water pollutants. Nine villages, built one above the other, shared the same water supply that flowed in a channel down the mountain. This water served every purpose: drinking and cooking, irrigation of crops, bathing, washing utensils and clothes, as a latrine, and as a basin for catching manure-saturated runoff water from cultivated fields.

While the water was relatively clean at the top of the mountain, as it flowed downward it gradually filled with organic pollutants so that the lower a village was situated the more polluted the water and the greater the incidence of goiters. It would be hard to find a cause of goiter among the people in these nine villages other than the amount of pollution in their water supply, since the incidence of goiter in each village correlated directly with the degree of pollution in the water they used.

In the United States there isn't a problem with organic water pollutants, since chlorine, a poisonous gas added to the water supply, kills off the bacteria that live off organic waste. There is no mineral, however, that neutralizes the toxic chemicals that have infiltrated the groundwater tables. Examples of water contamination by chemical wastes are resorcinol and dihydroxol, by-products of coal-mining operations in Kentucky. These have been discovered in the water supplies in towns in the Appalachian Mountains, where there is a high incidence of goiter, especially among children. Fluoridated water is also an inhibitor of thyroid function. Because the thyroid absorbs waterborne pollutants so easily, it's difficult to maintain normal thyroid function unless water used for drinking and cooking has been distilled or comes from underground springs that are tested regularly.

There isn't a mental or physical health problem in existence that can't be caused by an underactive thyroid—and therefore not one that can't be improved by normalizing thyroid function. The prime factor in maintaining a normal thyroid is the original source of energy that maintains every living thing on earth: direct sunlight, which is converted into chemical energy (ATP).

ATP is imbedded in the glucose molecules of the food we eat. It provides the raw material for cellular respiration. We obtain a supply of chemical energy when we eat, say, a banana. After it is digested, some of the glucose molecules in the banana are carried by the bloodstream to the mitochondria in the cells, where they are split up to release their energy. This chemical energy is converted to heat energy. But for this respiratory process to take place, red light, the longest light wave of the sun, must be present.

Gaining entry into the body through the eyes and skin, the red spectrum rays of sunlight are carried by the blood to the pineal gland. The pigment in the pineal absorbs it, just as light is absorbed into the chlorophyll pigment in the chloroplasts in leaves for the production of glucose.

There are still relatively unpolluted areas in the mountains and national parks in the United States where you can expose your body to a few weeks of good quality sunlight a year—the most important factor in the body's ability to generate energy.

CHAPTER 5

CARDIOVASCULAR DISEASE

Sam, my colleague at City College, born and raised on the African coast of Ghana, had a father who died at the age of 103 in full possession of his mental faculties. Sam believed he had inherited his father's longevity genes, since in looks and mind-set he was his carbon copy. His father, however, unlike Sam, had eaten healthy foods all his life. His dietary staple was fish that he ate right after he had caught and cleaned it, yams and cassava he dug up from the earth and threw into the fire minutes before he devoured them, and coconut milk he drank straight from the shell as soon as he got up in the morning. He sprinkled his food with what is considered the best salt in the world—mineral rich, reddish colored, and sweet tasting, it is raked up from the shoreline of the Ghana coast. Sam, on the other hand, having immigrated to the United States as a young man, had eaten processed foods most of his life. Now at age 86 his chances of living to be as old as his father were slim, since he was suffering from hardening of the arteries, a disease unknown among Ghanans—despite their high intake of salt.

I recommended to Sam that he change his diet instead of having an angioplasty, but he followed his doctors' advice and went ahead with the operation. In this procedure, a balloon is threaded through the arteries to the heart and expanded. After clearing away the plaque blocking the arteries, the surgeon implants a stent to keep the artery open, thus assuring the maximum flow of blood. The operation appeared at first to be a success. With his arteries cleared, Sam's chest pains went away and the increased flow of blood through the widened arteries now carried a sufficient supply of oxygen to the cells for the production of energy. Once again full of vigor, Sam no longer swayed and tottered when he walked, and his voice lost the gravelly sound typical of people with advanced heart disease.

Sam's return to health, however, was short-lived. The first symptom indicating his cardiovascular problems had returned was the slowing of his heartbeat. This is typically caused by an increase in estrogen (a sign that his testosterone levels had become deficient). Too much estrogen in the blood causes the veins carrying blood back to the heat to expand too much. This delays the return of the blood to the heart with the result that the heartbeat slows its pace. Within six months the inside walls of his arteries were once again encrusted with calcified plaque.

Reduce Acidic Waste to Revive Thyroid Function

Allergy-causing foods, inappropriate diet, and heavy metal accumulation create acidic waste. Circulating in the blood, this waste can lodge in the capillaries near the thyroid, blocking the flow of tyrosine (an amino acid) and iodine, the raw materials that go into the thyroid's production of thyroxin (T4). Acidic wastes can also clog the liver. This further reduces energy production, since the liver is responsible for converting T4 to the active T3.

Toxic waste in the blood also throws hormone levels out of balance. By elevating estrogen, it lowers progesterone, the hormone that is "thyroid friendly." Detoxification of the liver with vitamins E and C, and avoidance of junk food and foods your digestive system can't handle, heals the liver and restores its ability to convert T4 into its active form (T3).

What's Wrong with a High-Protein, Low-Carbohydrate Diet

Many people who want to lose weight look for the silver bullet that doesn't demand too much sacrifice but still guarantees weight loss. This is usually a diet that prohibits some foods while allowing unrestricted consumption of others. For example, one diet that was popular in the 1950s was all the bananas and ice cream you could eat but nothing else. This was a one-week diet. Another allows hardly any fat but the unrestricted consumption of carbohydrates. Such diets are appealing because they promise relief from ravenous hunger by allowing the dieter to pig out on one or two foods.

The most popular diet since it first appeared in England in 1860, in William Banting's book, Letter on Corpulence, and more recently in Dr. Robert C. Atkins's New Diet Revolution, is the high-protein, high-fat, low-carbohydrate diet. Its popularity is understandable because it takes weight off relatively easily, and eating lots of meats seems to lessen the hunger pangs that drive many people to binge eating—at least in the beginning.

But if the objective in losing weight is to improve health, that should be the driving force behind the choice of diet. The high-protein, low-carbohydrate diet does not fulfill that objective, because it is unbalanced. Eating so little starch deprives the body of glucose, its primary source of fuel, while eating too much meat threatens the body's mineral reserves. Excessive phosphate levels in meat can remove calcium and magnesium from the teeth and bones. Another danger to the body's supply of alkaline minerals is blood nitrogen urea from the breakdown of meat. Too much meat in the diet produces excessively high urea levels that the kidneys excrete along with magnesium and calcium.

Shifting viewpoints of the medical establishment as to what constitutes a healthy meal, as well as trendiness in diets, has made us lose sight of what used to be the axiom of nutritionists and doctors: the balanced meal made up of meat, potatoes, vegetables, and a lettuce and tomato salad. Indigenous cultures were not so quick to forget the knowledge of good nutrition passed on to them by their ancestors.

In most tribal societies in Africa, including both meat and starches in every meal was a time-honored tradition because it reflected the social structure of the clan. For example, among the Kaguru of central Tanzania a meal was said to be made up of both ugali (starches such as maize, millet, rice, plantain, and cassava) and nyama (stew meat). Only when nyama was not available did mboga (vegetables) take its place. Ugali represented the feminine gender because it was cultivated by women, while nyama was masculine because it was obtained by men's work as herdsmen and hunters. The well-balanced diets of these preindustrial cultures prevented obesity because they did not produce excessive levels of fatty acid wastes that build up layers of fat in the body.

Fighting Obesity with Acid-Alkaline Balance

The morbidly obese have unbalanced biochemistry. For many in this category hunger is not satisfied even when the stomach is filled. There are people who fall into the morbidly obese category even though they are moderate eaters.

Cheryl fit into the latter category. She was seventeen years old at the time I met her, weighed 350 pounds, and was five feet, six inches tall. Cheryl's mother showed me her medical records. Physical examinations by an endocrinologist, which included blood tests every year since she was twelve, failed to show any abnormalities in glandular function, blood lipid levels, or blood pressure. Nevertheless, Cheryl had some symptoms of ill health such as migraine headaches, depression, and swollen ankles and feet.

A ravenous appetite, however, was not one of her problems. At times she went all day without eating because she wasn't hungry. Her one liking was for sweets, and she ate two chocolate candy bars at a time once or twice a week, hardly enough to account for being two hundred pounds overweight. I believed Cheryl when she said she was not addicted to sweets, because the favorite marzipan cake her mother made her for her seventeenth birthday was practically intact one week later. Considering the small quantities of food Cheryl ate—her mother actually worried because she was hardly ever hungry—it was obvious she was not burning up her excess body fat. Her body shape was partly responsible. She had been chubby as a little girl, but before adolescence the fat was concentrated around her hips and thighs. As she put on the pounds, the fat crept up into her abdomen and chest. Excess fat in these regions is broken down and released into the bloodstream more quickly than the fat in the lower part of the body. This can lead to heart disease and liver damage.

It was essential for the sake of her health that Cheryl take off the excess layers of fat around the chest and abdomen. At my suggestion, she placed three five-by-twelve-inch magnetic pads over her chest and abdomen at night when she went to bed. Magnetic energy is a useful adjunct in a weight-loss program, because the negative charge of the magnets helps the growth hormone pull fat out of the fat cells. Happily, the removed fat is not deposited elsewhere. Not only do the chest and abdomen areas flatten out, weight typically drops by fifteen to twenty pounds. After about two months Cheryl's chest and upper abdomen were protruding less and she had taken off ten pounds.

Cheryl's rotund shape was not only dangerous to her health; it also made it very difficult for her to burn up fat. To generate additional energy for the purpose of losing weight, she took two teaspoons of coconut oil a day. At room temperature the oil is a solid, white block because it is supersaturated, but unlike meat and some dairy fats, coconut oil is not converted into cholesterol. Nor does it add to the stores of body fat. Being made up of medium chains of fatty acids, it gets burned up quickly. At the end of three months Cheryl had lost twenty pounds. This weight loss seems insignificant in relation to Cheryl's total weight, but it reduced the swelling in her ankles and feet.

To further raise Cheryl's energy level, with her doctor's approval I had her take some thyroid extract even though her thyroid function tested normal. The thyroid supplement raised her body temperature slightly above the normal 98.6 degrees. This caused her body to produce more energy than normal, and she burned off twenty more pounds of fat.

An increase in the production of energy is not much benefit if it isn't transported to wherever it is needed in the body, so Cheryl took 50 mg of CoQ-10 twice a day. But CoQ-10 did not cause further weight loss, probably because Cheryl's energy distribution system was normal. Cheryl melted away another fifteen pounds after she started playing badminton with her father for two hours, three times a week.

The weight that Cheryl lost as a result of these measures alleviated most of her health problems. While she still has migraine headaches, she no longer gets a blind spot in the center of her visual field during an attack, and her depressed moods occur less often. Cheryl's weight stabilized around 220 pounds—not enough weight loss for her to leave the morbidly obese category behind, but enough to make her feel—and look—much better. That was two years ago. Cheryl has maintained her weight loss.

Thyroid Problems

Sunlight is the stimulus that makes it possible for the thyroid to regulate the production of energy in the body. The stage is set for this assembly-line process when the first rays of sunlight in the morning are absorbed into the pigment of the brain's pineal gland. This act signals the pineal—the regulator of the sleeping-waking cycle of the body—to pass on the message via the pituitary gland to the thyroid that it must release additional thyroxin (T4) for the production of more energy. T4 flows through the bloodstream to the cells and delivers the message. (Before T4 can deliver this message, it must be converted by the liver into T3.) With the increased flow of energy to the organ systems, their functions speed up. This enables man to begin his daily struggle for existence.

The many diseases associated with deficient energy—cancer, hardening of the arteries, arthritis, diabetes, and obesity—make clear that a lack of energy because of a low-functioning thyroid can cut short our struggle for existence while we are still in our prime.

Testing for Underactive Thyroid

The basal thermometer test is a good way to start measuring your thyroid activity. Take your temperature with an old-fashioned mercury thermometer. It's the only reliable thermometer device. Place under the tongue or under your arm for seven to ten minutes three or four times a day. Upon waking before you get out of bed your temperature should be around 98 degrees; at midmorning after you've had breakfast and been up and around for a while, it should be normal—98.6 degrees. This temperature should be maintained until early evening when it begins to drop to around 98 degrees. Any temperature reading below these numbers indicates an underactive thyroid. When you're on thyroid medication and your temperature normalizes without causing an increase in the heart rate or pulse, you know you're taking enough medication to maintain normal thyroid function.

You can get an idea of whether foods depress your thyroid function by taking your temperature a half hour after eating a single food and then one hour after that. (This shouldn't be confused with the pulse test.) A below-normal temperature after eating a single food item is a pretty good indication of a food allergy. Drinking three cups of tea caused my temperature to fall by about one degree; after six cups of tea it dropped an additional degree. When I drink only one cup of tea, my 98.5 temperature remains steady.

The basal thermometer test may be the best overall test for hypothyroidism, because it measures what is most critical—the amount of energy generated inside the cell. However, there are other factors responsible for slow thyroid activity that should be measured. Most medical doctors rely solely on the TSH test to measure thyroid function. But you should take the following thyroid tests because each one tests something different: free T4, free T3, reverse T3, total T4, and total T3, as well as the thyroglobulin antibodies (TGA) test.

A thyroid test doctors rarely give is the reverse T3, probably because elevated reverse T3 is not a common cause of hypothyroidism. While regular T3 tells the energy-producing mitochondria in the cells how much energy to produce, reverse T3 blocks the regular T3 from entering the cells, with the result that energy production decreases.

The reverse T3 blocks energy production when there is too little intake of food. Thus in times of famine when there is not enough glucose or fat in the body, reverse T3 levels rise in order to lower energy production so that body fat and glucose are conserved.

When food becomes plentiful, reverse T3 blood levels drop far below that of regular T3, because with the intake of enough food there is no need to conserve body fuel. If despite the fact that you are eating enough, and your regular T3 level is normal, you still have the symptoms of an underactive thyroid, it may be because your reverse T3 levels are too high.

Why do a few individuals, although having plenty to eat, nevertheless have high levels of reverse T3? Dr. Richard Cordaro, a chiropractor and nutritionist in New York City, has found that nearly all individuals with excessive levels of reverse T3 suffer from heavy metal accumulation. Cordaro says that by removing the cadmium, mercury, lead, and other heavy metals from the body, reverse T3 levels are lowered and symptoms of hypothyroidism lessen or disappear altogether.

A dependable method for detecting heavy metal levels in the blood is the chelation test. Amino acids are injected into the blood where they bond with heavy metal molecules and are eliminated through the urine. After an injection, the urine is monitored for heavy metals over the next six hours.

You can't assume, because all the tests you take point to low thyroid function, that the trouble originates with the thyroid. It's possible that the parathyroid, the gland that regulates blood calcium levels, is responsible. If a patient has a problem with the parathyroid, it's a sign that thyroid function is also not normal, and the reverse is equally true.So, whether a patient comes to him with a thyroid or a parathyroid problem, Cordaro treats both glands.

An underactive thyroid can also be due to a deficiency of progesterone. Have your progesterone levels tested; if they are too low, ask your doctor to prescribe a natural progesterone cream or progesterone supplements

Elevated Blood Pressure Can Indicate a Low-Functioning Thyroid

If you're fifty or older, you can get a pretty good idea of how well your thyroid is functioning by taking your blood pressure. In my experience, when blood pressure is elevated, body temperature tends to be below normal, indicating that toxic debris from inappropriate food and heavy metals have raised the blood pressure by slowing down thyroid function. Monitoring your body temperature and your blood pressure to find out what foods are incompatible with your metabolism and then avoiding them is the most effective way to maintain normal thyroid function and good overall health.

It's hard to imagine that anyone age fifty or older who has both normal thyroid function and normal blood pressure could be suffering from any sort of degenerative illness. In older people, acidic waste from bad diet has already lowered thyroid function and raised blood pressure. Various studies indicate that anywhere from 50 to 90 percent of the population has a thyroid insufficiency.

If these figures were broken down by age, I'm sure it would show that nearly 100 percent of those over the age of fifty have an underactive thyroid—and that those who don't have a hyperactive thyroid! Individuals in their twenties, thirties, and sometimes even in their forties can eat junk food and still have normal thyroid function because they have enough enzymes to neutralize excessive levels of acid waste which interfere with thyroid function. But by late middle age some enzyme-producing glands have worn out from overwork.

Chapter Six

Alkaline Diets recipe

Almond-Quinoa Muffins

Servings: 12. Preparation time: 15 minutes. Cooking time: 15 to 18 minutes

Quinoa gives these muffins a bit of austerity, reminiscent of poppy seed muffins. It also adds a ton of protein to keep you energized throughout the day. This is not a very sweet muffin, it is a good choice when you don't want something too sweet but not salty. As with other muffin recipes, use a sprayed liner to keep the muffins from sticking out.

Recipe Tips: If you want to make your muffins a bit sweeter, add a packet of stevia in the batter and mix well.

Ingredients

- Cooking spray
- 1 cup vanilla almond milk
- ¼ cup of applesauce
- 1 tablespoon flax seeds
- 1 vanilla bean, cut longitudinally and shave off the seeds
- 1¼ cup coconut flour
- ¼ cup almond flour
- 1½ teaspoons baking powder
- ½ teaspoon sea salt
- ½ teaspoon ground cinnamon
- 1¼ cup cooked quinoa

Preparations

1.Preheat the oven to 350 ° F.

2. Line the muffin pan with paper lining and spray the lining with a cooking spray.

3. In a food processor, add almond milk, applesauce, flax seeds, and vanilla seeds. Blend until smooth.

4. In a medium bowl, combine coconut flour, almond flour, baking powder, salt, and cinnamon powder. These dry ingredients are added to a food processor and pulsed until a batter is formed.

5. Add quinoa and mix until completely mixed.

6. Use an ice cream scoop to oop the batter into a lined muffin pan and fill it with two-thirds.

7. Put the pan in a preheated oven and bake for 15 to 18 minutes, or until the inserted toothpick is clean.

8. Serve.

____

Per Serving (1 Meal): Calories: 170 / Total Fat: 6.1G / Carbohydrates: 24.9G / Fiber: 2.3G / Protein: 4.5G

Cauliflower Popcorn

Servings: 4. Preparation time: 10 minutes. Cooking time: 30 minutes

Nothing is more fun than watching a good movie and a bowl of popcorn. But since corn is on the "taboo" list, what do you do? Try a recipe that uses roasted broccoli instead of popcorn. Sprinkle with garlic powder, paprika or nutritious yeast.

Recipe Tips: Do not use frozen broccoli for this recipe. It's too wet.

Ingredients

- 1 cauliflower head, divided into small flowers
- 3 tablespoons coconut oil
- 1 teaspoon sea salt

Preparations

1.Preheat the oven to 400 ° F.

2. In a large bowl, mix cauliflower, coconut oil, and salt.

3. Transfer the cauliflower to a baking sheet and spread it evenly into a single layer.

4. Bake the slices in a preheated oven for about 30 minutes until golden brown and slightly crispy.

Per serving (approximately 1 cup): Calories: 107 / Total Fat: 10.3G / Carbohydrate: 3.5G / Fiber: 1.7G / Protein: 1.3G

Banana Nut Bread Smoothie

Serves: 1. Prep time: 2 minutes

Fresh vanilla beans add a nice flavor without the added sugar or alcohol found in vanilla extract. They're available in the spice section of many grocery stores. To prepare them, use a sharp knife to slice open the pod lengthwise and scrape the contents of the pod (the black seeds) into your recipe.

Recipe Tip Use a frozen banana and skip the ice cubes for a creamier treat. Or, use almond milk or coconut milk and skip the water.

Ingredients

- 1 cup filtered water
- 1 medium banana, peeled
- ¼ cup raw almonds
- ½ teaspoon cinnamon
- ¼ teaspoon nutmeg
- 1 whole vanilla bean, split lengthwise and seeds scraped out
- ½ cup ice cubes

Preparations

1. To a blender, add the water, banana, almonds, cinnamon, nutmeg, vanilla bean seeds, and ice.

2. Blend until smooth.

3. Serve in a tall glass.

PER SERVING: CALORIES: 254 / TOTAL FAT: 12.1G / CARBOHYDRATES: 33.4G / FIBER: 7.2G / PROTEIN: 6.3G

Banana Muffins

Servings: 12. Preparation time: 5 minutes. Cooking time: 15 to 18 minutes

These muffins are made from almond butter, which is found in most markets. Make sure the brand you get is free of added sugar or oil. In addition, use muffin liners sprayed with cooking spray so they can come out of the pan more easily. Freeze any leftovers (if any!) For quick, healthy snacks

The recipe suggests peeling and freezing bananas when they start to ripen. You can use them in smoothies or banana "ice cream", but you can also use them in muffin recipes. They are a bit mushy, but because they are mixed together, it doesn't matter.

Ingredients

- Cooking spray
- 2 ripe bananas
- 1 cup date
- ½ cup toasted buttered almond butter
- ½ cup coconut flour
- ¼ cup of melted coconut oil
- 2 teaspoons baking soda
- ½ teaspoon sea salt
- 1 vanilla bean, cut longitudinally and shave off the seeds

Preparations

1.Preheat the oven to 350 ° F.

2. Line the muffin pan with paper lining and spray the lining with a cooking spray.

3. In a food processor, add bananas and dates, and stir well.

4. Add almond butter, coconut flour, coconut oil, baking soda, salt and vanilla seeds to the processor and pulse until a thick batter is formed.

5. Use an ice cream spoon to oop the batter into a lined muffin jar and fill it with two-thirds.

6. Place the muffins in a preheated oven and bake for 15 to 18 minutes, or until the toothpick inserted in the muffins is clean.

7. serve.

____

Per Serving (1 Serving): Calories: 181 / Total Fat: 10.1 g / Carbohydrates: 21.7.4 g / Fiber: 2.6 g / Protein: 3.8 g

Orange, Peach, Kale Smoothie

Serve: 1. Preparation time: 10 minutes

The most time consuming part of this delicious recipe is peeled oranges. Because it's not long, it's a good choice for those busy mornings when you rush out of the door and want to grab something quickly. For faster smoothies, use frozen peaches. Just mix and start!

Recipe Tip If you can't find fresh peaches, freeze them. If there are only peaches in the can, drain and rinse before using.

Ingredients

- 1 orange, peeled and seeded
- 1 medium peach, peeled and sliced
- 1 cup chopped kale
- 8 ounces filtered water

Preparations

1. In a blender, add oranges, peaches, kale and water.

2. Handle until smooth.

3. Put it in a tall glass.

____

Per Serving: Calories: 158 / Total Fat: 0.05G / Carbohydrate: 38G / Fiber: 6.9G / Protein: 4.6G

Mango, Papaya, Raspberry Smoothie

Servings: 1 Preparation time: 2 minutes

Mango is a very good frozen fruit. This is a good thing because you can eat tropical fruit smoothies at any time of the year. Papaya is rich in vitamin C, which makes it ideal for fighting colds or other infections (avoid scurvy if you are a pirate). To add flavor, spread different fruits in the glass instead of mixing them together.

Recipe Tip: You can find frozen mangoes and other frozen fruits in your local market. If the smoothie is too thick after mixing, add water as needed.

Ingredients

- ¼ cup of raspberries
- ¾ cup frozen mango slices
- ½ medium papaya, seeded and chopped

Preparations

1. In a blender, add raspberries, mango and papaya.

2. Process until smooth.

3. Place in a tall glass.

____

Per Serving: Calories: 153 / Total Fat: 0.06G / Carbohydrates: 39.7G / Fiber: 6.7G / Protein: 2.1G

Basic Green Smoothie

Servings: 1. Preparation time: 2 minutes

No need to worry about green shakes. If you follow the basic formula, it really is delicious. To make a simple, healthy, and delicious green smoothie, mix a glass of leafy vegetables, a glass of liquid base, and a glass of fruit. Try this primer.

Recipe Tips: Feel free to use any fruit you like instead of peaches. Avoid blueberries as they are on the "No Entry" list.

Ingredients

- 1 cup spinach
- 1 cup unsweetened coconut milk
- 1 cup frozen cut peaches

1. In a blender, add spinach, coconut milk and peaches.

2. Handle until smooth.

3. Put it in a tall glass.

____

Per Serving: Calories: 230 / Total Fat: 6G / Carbohydrates: 43.5G / Fiber: 5.8G / Protein: 4.9G

Cucumber Soup

Servings: 1. Preparation time: 5 minutes

This cool cucumber smoothie is perfect for those hot days who don't want to heat the kitchen. The combination of avocado and cucumber is classic. This delicious smoothie is rich in nutrition and taste, and it is also alkaline!

Recipe Tips: Add a little paprika to heat.

Ingredients

- 1 cup peeled and diced cucumber
- ½ avocado
- ½ cup cold water
- ½ cup ice cubes
- Pinch garlic powder
- A handful of sea salt

Preparations

1. In a blender, add cucumber, avocado, water, ice, garlic powder and sea salt.

2. Process until the required consistency is achieved.

3. Put it in a tall glass.

____

Per serving: Calories: 221 / Total fat: 19.7G / Carbohydrates: 12.4G / Fiber: 7.2G / Protein: 2.6G

Baked Grapefruit

Servings: 1. Preparation time: 15 minutes. Cooking time: 15 minutes

Grapefruits are great at any temperature, but they are particularly good at baking. This vitamin C-rich fruit is rich in fiber and nutrients. After baking, brown sugar or maple syrup is usually sprinkled, but this version uses grated coconut instead. Make a hot breakfast on cold days.

Recipe Tips: Ruby Red is a grapefruit that is sweeter than other types of grapefruit. If you don't like grapefruit, try Ruby Red first.

Ingredients

- 1 grapefruit, halved
- 2 tablespoons grated unsweetened coconut

Preparations

1. Preheat the oven to 350 ° F.

2. Put the two halves of grapefruit on a foil-lined baking sheet. Put one tablespoon of coconut on top of each half.

3. Place the pan in a preheated oven and bake for 15 minutes, or until the coconut turns brown.

4. Cut the grapefruit in half and place it on a plate, then eat it with a spoon.

Per Serving: Calories: 86 / Total Fat: 0.07G / Carbohydrates: 11.9G / Fiber: 2.3G / Protein: 1.2G

Cherry-Chocolate Smoothie

Servings: 1. Preparation time: 2 minutes

Although regular cocoa powder is listed as a "taboo" when following an alkaline diet, cocoa powder processed in the Netherlands (a limited amount) is okay because it is processed in a way that produces an alkaline effect. Normal cocoa powder has a pH of 5.1 to 5.4; processed cocoa powder is more neutral with a pH of 6.8 to 8.1. And, because all cocoa powder is so rich, you can give you a chocolate flavor with just one touch, without adding extra acid to the recipe.

Recipe Tips:: Several popular chocolate brands produce cocoa powder processed in the Netherlands, so look in your local market or check out the Resources section to buy online.

Ingredients

- ½ cup frozen black cherries
- ¾ cup filtered water
- 1 teaspoon Dutch processed cocoa powder
- 1 packet of stevia (optional)

Preparations

1. In a blender, add cherries, water, cocoa powder and stevia (if used).

2. Processed to smooth

3. Place in a tall glass.

———————

Per Serving: Calories: 60 / Total Fat: 0.6G / Carbohydrates: 13.2G / Fiber: 1.8G / Protein: 0.5G

Mojito Smoothie

Servings: 1. Preparation time: 2 minutes

Although citrus fruits are acidic, once your body processes them, the result is alkalization. As a result, lime juice in this formula adds flavor but does not increase acidity. This drink is a great alternative to cocktails. It's rich in nutrients rather than calories.

The recipe suggests that you can substitute sweetness with lime. These little limes are less acidic than regular limes.

Ingredients

- 1 cup spinach
- 1 cup unsweetened coconut water
- 2 cups pineapple
- 2 tablespoons fresh mint leaves
- ½ lime juice

Preparations

1.In a blender, add spinach, coconut water, pineapple, mint leaves, and lime juice.

2. Handle until smooth.

3.Put it in a tall glass.

____

Per Serving: Calories: 241 / Total Fat: 1.5G / Carbohydrates: 60.4G / Fiber: 5.3G / Protein: 2.6G

Frosting Carrot Cake

Servings: 8. Preparation time: 15 minutes. Cooking time: 35 to 40 minutes

The cake is very moist due to the moisture in the pineapple and carrot. The secret is to make the batter into a cake and then add the pineapple to the center so that the juice is evenly mixed. When you turn the cake upside down, the cake forms a layer of filling, which automatically frosts. With this recipe, you can eat cake or eat it healthy!

Recipe Tips: If you don't crush pineapple by hand, you can process canned pineapples in a food processor and even use rings.

- Cooking spray
- ⅓ Coconut oil, add 3 tablespoons, melt and separate
- ½ cup grated carrot
- 1¼ cup almond flour
- 1½ teaspoons baking powder
- ¼ teaspoon sea salt
- 1 can (8 ounces) can squeeze the chopped juice of pineapple, drain the water, and retain the juice (about ¾ cup)
- ½ cup sliced sugar-free coconut
- ⅓ chopped almond cup

Preparations

1. Preheat the oven to 350 ° F.

2. Spray 8-inch round cake pans with cooking spray.

3. In a large bowl, mix combine cups of coconut oil and carrots.

4. In a medium bowl, sieve almond flour, baking powder, and salt. Add these dry ingredients to the carrot oil mixture, then add the retained pineapple juice. Mix thoroughly after each addition.

5. Sprinkle half of the batter in the prepared pan. Add the crushed pineapple evenly to the batter. Put the remaining cake batter on top.

6. In a small bowl, mix coconut, almonds, and the remaining 3 tablespoons of coconut oil. Sprinkle the almond mixture evenly over the cake.

7. Place the pan in a preheated oven and bake for 35 to 40 minutes, or until the cake tester is clean.

8. Carefully turn the pan upside down on the cake pan to reveal a perfectly shaped cake!

Per serving (⅛ of finished cake): Calories: 282 / Total fat: 26.6G / Carbohydrates: 10.3G / Fiber: 3.2G / Protein: 4.8G

Liquid Guacamole

Servings: 1. Preparation time: 2 minutes

The name of the recipe may take some time to get used to, but it tastes great! Avocado actually adds a delicious smooth texture that you can't get from anything else. Try it as an appetizer before a Mexican-style (alkaline food, of course) main meal.

Recipe Tips: Do not use this recipe if you are using the thyroid support program. In fact, avoid any recipes that include tomatoes or tomato products in the book.

Ingredients

- ½ avocado
- 1 cup spinach
- ¼ cup coriander
- 1 cup of fresh tomato juice
- Pinch garlic powder
- A handful of sea salt
- Pinch pepper
- ½ cup cherry tomatoes
- ½ cup diced cucumber

Preparations

1.In the blender, add avocado, spinach, parsley, tomato juice, garlic powder, salt and pepper.

2.Mix until smooth.

3.Add cherry tomatoes and cucumbers and mix until small pieces remain.

4.Put it in a tall glass.

____

Per Serving: Calories: 274 / Total Fat: 20.1G / Carbohydrates: 24.8G / Fiber: 9.5G / Protein: 5.6G

Baby Potato Home Fries

Servings: 2. Preparation time: 5 minutes. Cooking time: 20 minutes

Who needs a high-fat, high-sodium restaurant version of home fries? Instead, this healthy version uses baby white potatoes and a non-stick pan to give you all the flavors without the side effects of acids. If you have leftovers, you can cool them to make a potato salad. Breakfast or lunch!

Recipe Tips: You can also use small sweet potatoes in this recipe. It is best to avoid tan potatoes that are commonly used for baking because they contain a lot of starch.

Ingredients

- 4 medium-sized baby white potatoes
- 2 ounces vegetable soup
- ½ sweet white onion, chopped
- 1 red bell pepper, deseeded and diced
- ½ cup sliced mushrooms
- 1 teaspoon sea salt
- 1 teaspoon garlic powder

Preparations

1.In a safe microwave safe bowl, microwave the potatoes for 4 minutes, or until softened.

2.In a large non-stick pan over medium heat, add broth, onion and red bell pepper. Fry the vegetables for about 5 minutes, or until softened.

3.While the onions and peppers are cooked, cut the potatoes in half.

4.Add potatoes, mushrooms, salt, and garlic powder to a frying pan. Stir and mix. Cook for about 10 minutes, or until the potatoes are crispy

5. Serve when warm.

____

Per Serving (1 cup): Calories: 337 / Total Fat: 0.8G / Carbohydrates: 74.8G / Fiber: 12.4G / Protein: 9.3G

Brown Rice Porridge

Servings: 6. Preparation time: 5 minutes. Cooking time: 5 minutes

Brown rice and almond milk replace the white rice and milk traditionally found in this English-style breakfast. Feel free to add the fruit on hand. Banana and a bit of cinnamon will make it plump. Cherries and papaya will make it tropical. If the porridge is too thick, add a little coconut or almond milk before serving.

Recipe Tips: You can buy brown rice cereal on the market. In this recipe, replacing it with regular brown rice can make this alkaline-friendly dish faster and easier.

Ingredients

- 3 cups brown rice
- 1 cup almond milk
- 1 packet stevia

Preparations

1.In a medium pot, mix brown rice with almond milk. Cook over medium heat for 5 minutes and keep stirring until the mixture thickens and becomes milky.

2. Remove from the fire. Stir the stevia.

3. Divide into 6 bowls.

____

Per Serving (1/2 cup): Calories: 236 / Total Fat: 1.8G /
Carbohydrates: 48.3G / Fiber: 3.6G / Protein: 7G

Breakfast Parfait

Servings: 2. Preparation time: 10 minutes

This version of the parfait makes it easy to wonder why you have never done this before. Instead of yogurt or whipped cream, this recipe requires coconut whipped cream (here).

Recipe Tips: Feel free to exchange any fruit you like. Boldly add things like pumpkin or sweet potatoes!

Ingredients

- ¼ cup strawberry slices
- ¼ cup blackberry
- ¼ cup sliced raspberries
- ¼ cup of cut peaches
- 1 cup coconut cream (here)

Preparations

1.In a large transparent glass, put 2 tablespoons of strawberries and top it with 2 tablespoons of whipped cream. Add 2 tablespoons of blackberries and 2 tablespoons of whipped cream. Continue with 2 tablespoons of raspberries and 2 tablespoons of whipped cream. Finally add 2 tablespoons of peaches and 2 tablespoons of whipped cream.

2.Repeat the remaining ingredients in the second cup.

3.Launch immediately.

____

Per serving (½ cup of fruit and ½ cup of coconut cream):
Calories: 120 / Total Fat: 10G / Carbohydrates: 4G / Fiber: 6.3G
/ Protein: 1.7G

Sweet Potato Waffles With Applesauce

Servings: 4. Preparation time: 15 minutes. Cooking time: 5 to 7 minutes

This recipe may just become your new habit on Sunday morning. These waffles (or pancakes, without waffle iron nuggets) are so healthy and delicious that you won't even miss the sour milk you usually eat. Be careful when removing them from waffles, as they are very moist and brittle. If someone falls, eat it and call it "chef's bonus."

Recipe Tips: If you don't have applesauce, you can eat them with applesauce (here).

Ingredients

- 1¼ cup almond flour
- 2 teaspoons baking powder
- ½ teaspoon sea salt
- Dash Nutmeg
- Dash cinnamon
- ⅓ cup of coconut oil
- 1½ cups unsweetened coconut milk
- 1 cup mashed potatoes
- Cooking spray
- 1 cup unsweetened applesauce

Preparations

1. Preheat waffle iron.

2.In a large bowl, mix almond flour, baking powder, salt, nutmeg, and cinnamon.

3.In a medium bowl, stir coconut oil and coconut milk together until mixed.

4.Transfer the liquid ingredients to the bowl together with the dry ingredients. Stir until combined.

5. Pour the sweet potatoes gently into the batter, taking care not to stir too much.

6.Before making each waffle, spray the waffle iron with a cooking spray.

7. Make waffles in the direction indicated on the waffle iron.

8.Serve each waffle with 1/4 cup of applesauce.

____

Per serving (1 waffle plus 1/4 cup): Calories: 547 / Total Fat: 25G / Carbohydrates: 38G / Fiber: 16.9G / Protein: 14.6G

Spaghetti Squash Hash Browns

Servings: 2. Preparation time: 2 minutes. Cooking time: 10 minutes

Who needs high-fat, sour restaurant potato pancakes when you can make these delicious and nutritious foods at home? This recipe requires cooked spaghetti squash, so the day before making these noodles, simply place the spaghetti squash in the oven and bake (see note below). This way, the recipe is ready in just a few minutes. Serve with hearty breakfast sausages (here) and homemade tomato sauce (here). If you follow the Thyroid Support Program, just remember to skip ketchup.

Recipe Tips: Make sure you squeeze as much water as possible from the spaghetti squash to make it crispy.

Ingredients

- 2 cups cooked spaghetti squash
- ½ cup chopped onion
- 1 teaspoon garlic powder
- ½ teaspoon sea salt
- Cooking spray

Preparations

1.Use a paper towel to squeeze excess water from the spaghetti squash. Place pumpkins in a medium bowl. Add onion, garlic powder and salt. Blend mix.

2.Spray the frying pan in a non-stick pan with a cooking spray and heat over medium heat.

3.Add the pumpkin mixture to the pot. Cook for 5 minutes and leave as it is. Turn the potato cake with a spatula. It is also possible to spread the mixture. Cook for another 5 minutes or until the desired crispness is reached.

To bake pasta squash, cut the pumpkin in half lengthwise and shave off the seeds. Brush each half with 2 tablespoons of coconut oil and season with 1 teaspoon of sea salt. Cut the pumpkin in half and place it on a baking sheet with the side up and bake at 350 ° F for about 50 minutes, or until the fork is soft.

____

Per Serving (1 cup): Calories: 44 / Total Fat: 0.6G / Carbohydrates: 9.7G / Fiber: 0.6G / Protein: 0.9G

Pumpkin-Spice Quinoa Casserole

Servings: 6. Preparation time: 5 minutes. Cooking time: 15 minutes

This hearty casserole can be assembled the night before baking to make morning preparation easy. Quinoa is a protein powerhouse that adds nutty flavor. Pumpkin is rich in beta-carotene and fiber. Using cooked quinoa makes assembly easier. This breakfast will keep you busy all day.

Recipe Tips: You can actually heat this dish in the microwave to make it faster. Just place the mixture high in the microwave for 7 minutes, or until the pumpkin solidifies.

Ingredients

- Cooking spray
- 3 cups quinoa
- 1 can (15 ounces) pumpkin puree
- ½ glass of water
- 1 vanilla bean, cut longitudinally and shave off the seeds
- 1 teaspoon cinnamon
- ½ teaspoon nutmeg
- ½ teaspoon ginger powder
- ¼ teaspoon ground fresh ginger
- ¼ teaspoon sea salt

Preparations

1. Preheat the oven to 350 ° F.

2.Spray 4 cups of casserole and set aside.

3.In a medium bowl, stir together quinoa, pumpkin, water, vanilla seeds, cinnamon, nutmeg, ginger powder, fresh ginger, and salt.

4.Transfer the mixture to the prepared casserole. Bake for 15 minutes, or until golden brown with bubbles.

____

Per Serving (1 cup): Calories: 26 / Total Fat: 5G / Carbohydrates: 57.1G / Fiber: 7.7G / Protein: 12G

Breakfast Fajitas

Servings: 2. Preparation time: 5 minutes. Cooking time: 10 minutes

The staple of this restaurant can easily be used as a wonderful breakfast. This is a great option to take in healthy vegetables and fill your stomach to start your day. If you like, you can wrap these Mexican cabbages in lettuce leaves, but they are excellent, just use a fork to serve them hot from the frying pan.

Recipe Tips: have a source link in the Resources section for coconut flour tortillas. Wrap one around fajitas and enjoy a hearty breakfast.

Ingredients

- Cooking spray
- 1 bell pepper, any color, pitted, seeded and sliced
- 1 finely chopped onion, such as Vidalia
- 1 cup cooked broccoli floret
- ½ cup sliced mushrooms
- 1 cup cherry tomatoes, halved when large
- ½ cup sliced zucchini or other pumpkin
- 2 cloves of garlic, peeled and chopped
- 1 mexican roll, chopped (optional)
- 1 teaspoon sea salt
- ½ teaspoon cumin

- 2 tablespoons fresh coriander
- ½ lime juice
- Salsa Fresca (here), serving gourmet food

Preparations

1. Spray a large non-stick pan with a cooking spray and place it on medium heat.

2. Add bell pepper, onion, broccoli, mushrooms, tomatoes, zucchini, garlic, and jalapeno (if used). Cook and stir for about 7 minutes, or until the desired tenderness is reached.

3. Add salt, cumin and parsley and stir. Cook and stir for 3 minutes.

4. Remove from fire and add lime juice.

5. Separate between two plates and serve with Salsa Fresca.

Per Serving (1/2 servings of final formula): Calories: 86 / Total Fat: 0.07G / Carbohydrates: 17.4G / Fiber: 5.1G / Protein: 4.1G

Vegetable Chips

Servings: 4. Preparation time: 5 minutes. Cooking time: 20 minutes

These crispy potato chips are more flavorful and nutritious than traditional potato chips. And because they are grilled, not fried, they are fully compliant with alkaline dietary regulations. Serve with spinach artichoke dip (here) or healthy hummus (here). Feel free to use other root vegetables and do interesting experiments.

Recipe Tips: Add these fries with garlic powder, paprika, curry powder, or other alkaline seasonings to add flavor.

Ingredients

- 1 parsnip, peeled
- 1 large carrot, peeled
- 1 beet peeled
- 1 sweet potato peeled
- 1 teaspoon sea salt
- Cooking spray

Preparations

1.Preheat the oven to 375 ° F.

2.Use a food processor attachment, a mandolin or a food slicer to slice parsnips, carrots, beets and sweet potatoes. Lay the slices flat on a paper towel and sprinkle with salt. Cover with more paper towels and let stand for 15 minutes.

3.Absorb moisture on vegetable slices.

4.Spray the baking sheet with cooking spray.

5. Place a single layer of sliced vegetables on a baking sheet. Spray the vegetables with a cooking spray.

6.Place the flakes in a preheated oven and bake for about 20 minutes, or until crisp.

Per serving (¼ of final formula): Calories: 69 / Total Fat: 0.2G / Carbohydrate: 16.1G / Fiber: 3.5G / Protein: 1.4G

Sweet Potato Fries

Servings: 2. Preparation time: 10 minutes. Cooking time: 30 minutes

Sweet potato fries are all the rage these days. This is not surprising, since a potato contains more than twice the daily vitamin A content. These baked fries are simple and delicious, and you won't miss the fryer. To make changes, sprinkle them with garlic powder, paprika, nutritious yeast or stevia and cinnamon powder.

The recipe suggests a difference between sweet potatoes and yam. The flesh of sweet potatoes is orange, and the flesh of yam is white. Both are fried into delicious.

Ingredients

- 2 sweet potatoes, peeled and cut into fries
- Cooking spray
- 1 teaspoon sea salt

Preparations

1. Preheat the oven to 425 ° F.

2.Spray the baking sheet with cooking spray.

3.Place the fries on a thin plate. Wrap the fries with cooking spray and sprinkle with salt.

4.Place the flakes in a preheated oven for 15 minutes. Turn the fries over. Cook for another 15 minutes, or until crispy. Servings:.

____

Per serving (1/2 serving of final formula): Calories: 71 / Total Fat: 0.02G / Carbohydrates: 5.8G / Fiber: 0.3G / Protein: 2.1G

Pumpkin Drink

Servings: 1. Preparation time: 2 minutes

One of the first signs of autumn is the advent of pumpkin spices. With this recipe, you can have a traditional ice-blended pumpkin without using sour dairy, sugar and coffee ingredients. Instead, you replace it with fiber, antioxidants, minerals, and vitamins. It's so delicious you won't even miss the bad stuff.

Recipe Tips:: Make sure to use pumpkin puree (pure pumpkin) instead of "pumpkin pie filling". Pie fillings are filled with sugar and dairy products.

Ingredients

- ½ cup pumpkin puree
- 1 banana, frozen
- 1 cup unsweetened coconut milk
- 1 vanilla bean, cut longitudinally and shave off the seeds
- ¼ teaspoon cinnamon
- ⅛ teaspoon nutmeg
- Teaspoon five spice powder
- ½ cup ice cubes

Preparations

1. In a blender, add pumpkin, banana, coconut milk, vanilla seeds, cinnamon, nutmeg, allspice and ice.

2. Handle until smooth.

3. Put it in a tall glass.

____

Per Serving: Calories: 240 / Total Fat: 5.5G / Carbohydrates: 47.6G / Fiber: 7.6G / Protein: 3.6G

Santa's Ginger Snaps

Servings: 6. Preparation time: 10 minutes. Cooking time: 10 to 15 minutes

You think you probably won't buy alkaline-friendly cookies! Well, the ingredients for these snacks are on the "Go" list. These ginger slices are so tender and delicious that you don't want to share them with Santa. Serve with iced almond milk and feel like a kid again!

Recipe Tips: Do not use fresh ginger in this recipe. It does not mix well with the ingredients, leaving a lot of ginger in the cookies.

Ingredients

- ½ cup almond flour
- ⅓ cup of coconut flour
- ⅓ cup of coconut sugar
- 2 tbsp kudzu powder
- ½ teaspoon baking soda
- ½ teaspoon ginger powder
- ½ teaspoon cinnamon
- ¼ teaspoon sea salt
- ¼ teaspoon cloves
- ¼ cup coconut oil

- 3 tablespoons flax seeds, immersed in 3 tablespoons
  warm water

Preparations

1.Preheat the oven to 350 ° F.

2.Put parchment paper on the baking sheet.

3.In a large bowl, mix almond flour, coconut flour, coconut sugar, bamboo taro, baking soda, ginger, cinnamon powder, salt and cloves.

4.In a microwave-heatable bowl, heat the microwave to 30 seconds to melt the coconut oil. Mix it with the flaxseed mixture. Pour the coconut oil mixture with the dry ingredients into a bowl. Stir and mix. The dough has hardened.

5. Pick up the dough with a spoon and roll it into small balls by hand. Place the dough balls on a prepared baking sheet and press into a circular dish.

6.Place the flakes in a preheated oven and bake for 10 to 15 minutes, or until hardened.

7. Let cool before serving.

Per serving (2 cookies): Calories: 174 / Total fat: 10.4G / Carbohydrates: 17.2G / Fiber: 1.7G / Protein: 2.8G

Scout Cookies

Servings: 12. Preparation time: 30 minutes. Cooking time: 5 minutes, roasted coconut

This recipe is more complicated than the other recipes in this book. The advantage of this recipe is that it is the original recipe, which means it is not baked. Since the formula contains alkalized cocoa powder, these cookies make up a portion of your 20%. Freeze any leftovers to control these delicious and healthy foods.

This formulation shows that the use of potassium carbonate in Dutch processing neutralizes the high acidity of cocoa to pH 7. Find Dutch-processed cocoa in your local market or "source".

Ingredients

For cookie library

- 1 cup dried unsweetened shredded coconut
- 1 cup raw almonds
- 2 pinches of sea salt
- 2½ tablespoons melted coconut oil
- 1 packet stevia

For coconut caramel layer

- ½ cup unsweetened shredded coconut
- 8 Medjool dates

- 1 tablespoon water, add if needed

- 2 tablespoons coconut oil, melted

- Small amount of sea salt

For chocolate icing

- 4 tablespoons coconut oil, melted

- 1 packet stevia

- 4 tablespoons sugar-free

- Cocoa powder

Preparations

1.Place parchment paper on a baking sheet.

2.In a food processor, mix coconut for 60 seconds. Add almonds and salt and mix until they are ground. Incorporate coconut oil and stevia until a dough is formed.

3.Roll the dough between two sheets of wax paper to a thickness of 1/4 inch. Freeze the dough for 10 minutes, or until hardened.

4.Use a round cookie cutter to cut out 12 cookies. Place each cookie base on a baking sheet lined with parchment paper.

Make the coconut caramel layer:

1.Preheat the oven to 350 ° F.

2.Spread the coconut evenly on another baking sheet. Bake in a preheated oven for 5 minutes, taking care not to burn it. Remove and cool.

3.Add dates, water and coconut oil to the food processor. Mix together. Add salt and more water if needed. Continue mixing until the mixture resembles caramel. Add toasted coconut and mix together.

4.Spread an even layer of caramel-coconut mixture on each cookie base.

Making chocolate icing:

1.In a small bowl, mix coconut oil, stevia, and cocoa powder.

2.Spoon powdered sugar on 12 biscuits.

3. Refrigerate the cookies for 10 minutes before meals to allow the layers to solidify.

____

Per serving (1 cookie): Calories: 180 / Total Fat: 16.9G / Carbohydrates: 7.4G / Fiber: 2.3G / Protein: 2.2G

Spinach-Artichoke Dip

Servings: 6. Preparation time: 10 minutes. Cooking time: 20 minutes

The staple food of such parties and restaurants is usually made of fatty yoghurt. Usually so salty that you can only taste fat and salt-where are the vegetables? This version tastes creamy (without any dairy products!) And you can actually taste the delicious spinach and artichoke flavors. Rich in nutrition and taste, you may never eat another version again. If you follow the Thyroid Support Program, be sure not to disturb the tomatoes.

Recipe Tips: If you like, you can use frozen spinach in this recipe. Just make sure you squeeze out all the water.

Ingredients

- Cooking spray
- ¾ cup raw cashews
- ¾ cup unsweetened almond milk
- 2 tablespoons freshly squeezed lemon juice
- 1 clove garlic
- ¾ teaspoon sea salt
- 1 tablespoon nutritional yeast
- 2 cups artichoke hearts, frozen or canned with water instead of oil
- 2 cups baby spinach leaves

- 1 cup small tomatoes

Preparations

1.Preheat the oven to 425 ° F.

2.Spray the medium baking sheet with cooking spray.

3.In a blender, mix cashews, almond milk, lemon juice, garlic, salt and yeast. Blend until very smooth.

4.Add artichoke hearts, spinach and tomatoes to the blender. Pulses merge, but large chunks of vegetables remain.

5. Transfer the dipping sauce to the prepared baking sheet. Place the bowl in a preheated oven and bake for 20 minutes.

6.Remove from the oven, cool for 5 minutes, then heat.

____

Per Serving (¼ cup): Calories: 178 / Total Fat: 15.3G / Carbohydrates: 10.3G / Fiber: 2.3G / Protein: 4.4G

Healthy Hummus

Servings: 4. Preparation time: 5 minutes

Traditional hummus is already healthy. However, since chickpeas are one of the foods you should limit, this version adds some eggplant to add flavor while limiting beans. Doing so makes this recipe taste like a delicious combination of hummus and baba manna. To bake the eggplant, place it on a baking sheet and bake in an oven at 350 ° F for 30 minutes, or until softened.

Recipe Tips: If you are in the thyroid support program, omit the eggplant and add another cup of chickpeas.

Ingredients

- 1 cup chickpeas, canned or cooked
- 1 cup eggplant, roasted and peeled
- 1 clove garlic
- 1 tablespoon sesame oil
- 1 tablespoon freshly squeezed lemon juice
- 1 teaspoon sea salt
- Water for dilution

Preparations

In a food processor, mix chickpeas, eggplant, garlic, sesame oil, lemon juice and salt. Blend until creamy and smooth. If necessary, add water to form a creamy consistency.

––––––––––––––

Per serving (½ cup): Calories: 219 / Total Fat: 6.5G / Carbohydrates: 31.9G / Fiber: 9.5G / Protein: 9.9G

Chile-Lime Mango Slaw

Servings: 1. Preparation time: 5 minutes. Cooling time: 15 minutes

This dish is a twist on popular street food in Los Angeles and Mexico. Lime juice and a bit of paprika revitalize the sweet and crunchy mango. If jicama is unfamiliar, prepare for treatment. This mild, crunchy root is great as a snack or salad.

Recipe Tips: If you feel lazy, skip the skewers and add lime juice and paprika directly to the mango, core it and score it.

Ingredients

- 1 mango, peeled and cut into small pieces
- 1 cup sliced jicama
- 1 cup bell pepper flakes
- 1 lime juice
- 1 tablespoon paprika

Preparations

1.In a small bowl, add mango, bell pepper, and jicama.

2. Squeeze the lemon juice over the vegetables. Sprinkle with paprika.

3. Refrigerate for 15 minutes to blend and enjoy the flavors.

____

Per Serving: Calories: 201 / Total Fat: 1.3G / Carbohydrate: 50G / Fiber: 5G / Protein: 2.8G

Orange Healthy Smoothie

Servings: 1. Preparation time: 2 minutes

This smoothie reminds you of delicious orange frozen foods that are usually available in shopping malls. Without sugar and dairy products, you can enjoy this fresh milk smoothie anytime and still follow your diet plan. If your orange juice is not that sweet, you can add a pack of stevia. Like all smoothies in this chapter, make sure to drink immediately or the ingredients will start to separate.

Recipe Tips: If you don't have freshly squeezed orange juice, you can use it in a carton. Just make sure it's organic and doesn't add any sugar. Avoid the kind produced in re-concentrated concentrates.

Ingredients

- 6 ounces freshly squeezed orange juice
- 1 ounce unsweetened coconut milk
- 1 medium frozen banana, cut into pieces
- 1 vanilla bean, cut longitudinally and shave off the seeds
- 1 packet of stevia (optional)

Preparations

1. In a blender, add orange juice, coconut milk, banana, vanilla seeds, and stevia (if used).

2. Handle until smooth.

3. Put it in a tall glass.

____

Per Serving: Calories: 182 / Total Fat: 0.3G / Carbohydrates: 44G / Fiber: 3.8G / Protein: 2.3G

Tea Party Cucumber Sandwiches

Servings: 2. Preparation time: 10 minutes

Isn't the tea party fun? Unfortunately, afternoon tea is often an excuse for eating sugary and fatty foods. Instead, eat these breadless sandwiches with tea and some cookies in this book. You can enjoy a relaxing afternoon and know that you are supporting your health, so feel happy.

The recipe suggests that you can quickly cook asparagus in the microwave and then run in cold water to cool it.

Ingredients

- ½ cup healthy hummus (here)
- 1 cucumber, peeled and cut into 1 / 4-inch small circles
- 4 asparagus spears, trimmed, cooked, cooled and chopped

Preparations

1.Place 1 teaspoon of hummus on a cucumber circle. Add 1/2 teaspoon of asparagus on top. Pour the second cucumber on top. Carefully place the sandwich on a plate.

2.Repeat the remaining ingredients.

____

Per Serving (4 Sandwiches): Calories: 126 / Total Fat: 6.2G /
Carbohydrates: 14.4G / Fiber: 4.5G / Protein: 5.9G

Mango-Barbecue Sliders

Servings: 2. Preparation time: 5 minutes. Cooking time: 10 minutes

One thing many people will miss by following an alkaline diet is meat. Although this recipe does not contain any meat, it definitely provides a satisfying and hearty barbecue flavor. Bring this dish to an outdoor picnic and hear everyone say, "It looks great!" These are messy, so there are a lot of napkins on hand.

Recipe Tip If you don't have zucchini, substitute 1 cup of cooked and chopped spaghetti squash.

Ingredients

- 1 mango, peeled, pitted and cut into large pieces
- ¼ cup of homemade barbecue sauce (here)
- 1 zucchini, peeled and shredded
- 4 mushrooms mushroom cover, remove g

Preparations

1.Preheat the grill or baking tray on the stove to medium heat.

2.In a food processor, mango puree is made into puree. Add homemade barbecue sauce. Transfer the mixture to a medium-sized bowl. Add zucchini and mix well.

3.Fill half of the mango-zucchini mixture with a mushroom cap. Put another mushroom cap on top.

4.Repeat the remaining ingredients to make a second slider.

5. Place the sliders on the grill and cook for 10 minutes, or until the desired tenderness is reached.

6.Eat immediately.

———————

Per serving (1 slide step): Calories: 135 / Total fat: 0.6G / Carbohydrate: 32.2G / Fiber: 3.1G / Protein: 1.7G

Banana Candy Coins

Servings: 1. Preparation time: 2 minutes. Cooking time: 5 minutes

Sometimes you just want sweets and now you want them. With these delicious foods, you don't have to wait to bake a cake or a batch of cookies. You can eat sweets and help your health in 5 minutes! For this recipe, choose a sturdy banana.

Recipe Tips: Try making this recipe with plantain (banana's cousin is less sweet). These coins will be stronger and less sweet than coins made from bananas.

Ingredients

- 2 tablespoons chopped unsweetened coconut
- A handful of sea salt
- 2 tablespoons coconut oil
- 1 banana, peeled and cut into 1 / 4-inch thick slices

Preparations

1.On a plate, combine coconut and salt.

2.Melt coconut oil in a medium pot over medium heat.

3.Press each banana slice into the coconut mixture until covered.

4.Gently place each slice in heated coconut oil. Fry for 2 minutes, turn over, and continue cooking on the second side for 2 to 3 minutes.

5. Cool it a little, then heat it.

____

Per Serving: Calories: 171 / Total Fat: 6.3G / Carbohydrates: 28.4G / Fiber: 4.4G / Protein: 1.5G

The Breakup Bowl

Servings: 1. Preparation time: 5 minutes

Almost everyone happened. You get dumped don't let it ruin your healthy eating plan! Don't cry a pint of ice cream, but pour these sweet and healthy ingredients into a bowl to soothe your body and soul.

The recipe hints that you can add other fruits as needed. Frozen cherries and fresh strawberries are great choices.

Ingredients

- 2 bananas, peeled, sliced and frozen
- 2 tablespoons coconut milk
- 2 tablespoons sweetened strawberry jam
- 2 tablespoons grated unsweetened coconut
- 2 tablespoons chopped roasted almonds
- ¼ cup coconut cream

Preparations

1.In a food processor, place frozen bananas. Add coconut milk and mix until the consistency of the ice cream is reached. Transfer to a single bowl.

2.Add jam, coconut, toasted almonds and whipped cream to the banana.

3.Serve immediately.

____

Per Serving: Calories: 454 / Total Fat: 19.2G / Carbohydrates: 69.4G / Fiber: 9.6G / Protein: 6.9G

Snickerdoodle Cookies

Servings: 6. Preparation time: 10 minutes. Cooking time: 10 to 12 minutes

This recipe uses basic cookie ingredients and adds a delicious change to the theme. Feel free to try it by adding food to the Start list. Here, the classic Snickerdoodle sugar cookies have been reconstituted to have a strong vanilla flavour.

Ingredients

- ½ cup almond flour
- ⅓ cup of coconut flour
- ⅔ One cup of coconut sugar, divided
- 2 tbsp kudzu powder
- ½ teaspoon baking soda
- ¼ teaspoon sea salt
- 1 teaspoon cinnamon
- ¼ cup coconut oil
- 3 tablespoons flax seeds, immersed in 3 tablespoons warm water
- 1 vanilla bean, cut longitudinally and shave off the seeds

Preparations

1.Preheat the oven to 350 ° F.

2. Put parchment paper on the baking sheet.

3. In a large bowl, mix almond flour, coconut flour, cup of coconut sugar, kudzu flour, baking soda and salt together.

4. In a small bowl, add the remaining cup of coconut sugar and cinnamon powder. Stir and mix.

5. In a microwave-heatable bowl, heat the microwave to 30 seconds to melt the coconut oil. Add flax seed mixture and vanilla seeds. Stir and mix.

6. Mix the coconut oil mixture with the dry ingredients into a bowl. Blend mix. The dough has hardened.

7. Shape the dough into 1-inch balls by hand. Roll each dough ball into the reserved cinnamon sugar. Place them on prepared baking sheets spaced about 1.5 inches apart.

8. Place the baking sheet in a preheated oven and bake for 10 to 12 minutes, or until the top of the stove turns brown.

9. Cool on a wire rack and serve.

____

Per serving (2 cookies): Calories: 174 / Total fat: 10.4G / Carbohydrates: 17.2G / Fiber: 1.7G / Protein: 2.8G

Stuffed Peppers

Servings: 2. Preparation time: 5 minutes. Cooking time: 20 minutes

This quick and easy recipe also looks elegant. The vibrant pepper combined with the colors of vegetables and quinoa makes it look worth a taste. It is high in fiber, high in protein and delicious. Leftovers and leftovers are also a good lunch for work the next day.

Ingredients

- Cooking spray
- 1 teaspoon coconut oil
- ½ cup chopped vegetables, zucchini, carrots or broccoli
- 1 cup cooked quinoa
- 1 teaspoon garlic powder
- 1 teaspoon onion powder
- 1 teaspoon sea salt
- 2 seedless, seedless bell peppers; top removed and retained

Preparations

1.Preheat the oven to 350 ° F.

2.Apply a cooking spray to the baking sheet.

3.Add coconut oil and chopped vegetables to a medium pot over medium heat. Fry for 5 minutes, or until softened.

4.Add quinoa, garlic powder, onion powder and salt. Stir and mix.

5. Place each bell pepper vertically in the prepared pot. Add half of the quinoa vegetable mixture to each pepper. Put the reserved top on each pepper.

6.Cover the aluminum foil, place in a preheated oven, and bake for 15 minutes, or until the peppers are soft.

____

Per Serving (1 Pack Pepper): Calories: 213 / Total Fat: 5.1G / Carbohydrates: 34.8G / Fiber: 5.5G / Protein: 7.2G

White Sauce

Servings: 6. Preparation time: 5 minutes. Cooking time: 10 minutes

This is another staple sauce that covers almost everything. Ideal for use on vegetables and bowls. Like gravy, practice a little bit so you can make it right. Then, amaze your friends with this healthy sauce.

Recipe Tips:: Once you know the basics of the sauce, you can add various seasonings to it to make changes. Try adding basil or fresh rosemary, or use it for mushroom soup. The options are almost endless.

Ingredients

- 1 tablespoon coconut oil
- 3 tablespoons coconut flour
- 2¼ cup almond milk
- 1 teaspoon sea salt
- 1 teaspoon garlic powder
- 1 teaspoon onion powder

Preparations

1. In a saucepan over medium heat, gently heat the coconut oil. Don't let it overheat or the flour will burn immediately.

2. Add coconut flour and stir into a thick paste.

3. Add almond milk and bring to a boil. Boil for 2 minutes, then reduce heat.

4. Add salt, garlic powder and onion powder. simmer until thickened

5. Servings: is warm.

____

Per Serving (½ cup): Calories: 83 / Total Fat: 4.1G / Carbohydrates: 8.1G / Fiber: 0.5G / Protein: 3.5G

Curried Eggplant

Servings: 2. Preparation time: 5 minutes. Cooking time: 5 minutes

This incredible dish is both healthy and delicious. Making an eggplant by hand is a good idea because it is easy to make and you always have a meal in your hand for a light meal.

Ingredients

- 1 roasted eggplant, after cooling, remove the contents from the shell and keep
- 1 lemon juice
- 1 teaspoon sea salt
- 1 teaspoon sesame oil
- 1 teaspoon curry powder
- Water as needed
- Quinoa cooked for consumption (optional)

Preparations

1.In a food processor, mix eggplant, lemon juice, salt, sesame oil and curry powder together. Blend until smooth.

2.Place it in a small pot over medium heat and heat the eggplant mixture for about 5 minutes. If necessary, dilute with some water.

3.Served as is or on quinoa (if used).

To bake the eggplant, simply slice it, add a bit of sea salt, and bake in an oven at 300 ° F for about 30 minutes, or until it becomes soft. Alternatively, you can bake it whole as requested here, but depending on the size, it takes longer to cook until it is easily pierced with a sharp knife. Refrigerate in the refrigerator until use.

———————

Per serving (1/2 serving of final formula): Calories: 81 / Total Fat: 2.8G / Carbohydrates: 14.1G / Fiber: 8.4G / Protein: 2.4G

Sprouted Beans

Servings: 4. Preparation time: 3 to 4 days, depending on the type of beans

Germinating beans is one way to reduce their acidic effects and it's easy to do. You probably did this in elementary school. Just make enough so that you can eat it in a few days.

Recipe Tips:: If you don't want to run into all the trouble, you can buy sprouted beans at most health food stores. But hey, try it at least once!

Ingredients

- Selection of 1 cup dried beans
- ½ teaspoon sea salt

Preparations

1. Rinse the beans and soak them in enough water overnight to cover the salt and sea salt.

2. In the morning, drain the beans and rinse with a colander in a bowl or sink. Cover with beans.

3. Wash and drain the beans several times a day until the beans start to germinate. This takes 3 to 4 days, depending on the type of bean.

4. Store in the refrigerator for a day or two.

Per Serving (¼ serving final formula): Calories: 10 /
Carbohydrates: 2G / Fiber: 0.9G / Protein: 0.5G

Coconut Whipped Cream

Servings: 8. Preparation time: 15 minutes

This recipe will make you glad to have purchased this book. Seriously-isn't it whipped cream made from dairy products? The key to success here is to refrigerate a can of coconut milk overnight, so when you open it, the cream is on top of the can. Use only the solidified portion of coconut cream, not water.

The recipe suggests that whipped coconut milk takes longer than whipped cream. Be patient! Also, if you want to make it sweeter, use coconut sugar instead of stevia.

Ingredients

- 1 (13 ounces) whole fat unsweetened coconut milk, refrigerated
- 1 packet stevia
- 1 vanilla bean, cut longitudinally and shave off the seeds

Preparations

1. Open a jar of coconut milk. Use a spoon to oop out thick coconut milk fat. Put it in a large bowl. Beat with an egg beater or a hand mixer, just like regular butter until fluffy.

2. Add stevia and vanilla seeds and whipped for about a minute.

3. Use immediately or cover the refrigerator for one to two days.

____

Per Serving (¼ cup): Calories: 197 / Total Fat: 21.2G /
Carbohydrates: 2.8G / Fiber: 0.1G / Protein: 2G

Apple Butter

Servings: 24. Preparation time: 10 minutes. Cooking time: 3 hours

This is an excellent spread on any muffin in this recipe. It may take some time, but your entire house will smell like autumn. And rich in fiber and nutrients.

Recipe Tips:: This recipe can use apple cider instead of apple juice, but choose some unsweetened apple cider. Also, don't use cinnamon or spices in this recipe.

Ingredients

- 4 pounds apple peeled and cored and chopped
- 2 glasses of fresh apple juice
- 1 tablespoon freshly squeezed lemon juice
- 2 packets of stevia
- 1 teaspoon cinnamon
- 1 vanilla bean, cut longitudinally and shave off the seeds
- Pinch cloves

Preparations

1. In a large pot, combine apples, apple juice and lemon juice. Cook over low heat for an hour until softened. Remove from fire and cool slightly.

2. Use an immersion blender (or use your regular blender in batches) to cut the apple puree into fines.

3. Add stevia, cinnamon, vanilla seeds and cloves to the apple. Reheat the pot and cook for another 2 hours, stirring frequently.

4. Cool apple butter. Transfer to a closed container and refrigerate.

____

Per serving (2 tablespoons): Calories: 49 / Total fat: 0.2G / Carbohydrates: 12.9G / Fiber: 1.9G / Protein: 0.2G

The Asian Bowl

Servings: 1. Preparation time: 5 minutes

The standard way to make a good bowl is to layer cereals, beans, vegetables and seasonings. Of course, the recipes in this book only contain ingredients from the approved food list, so cereals are often replaced by another vegetable. The basis of this Asian bowl is chopped cabbage. If you want a warm bowl, fry the cabbage and carrots first.

Recipe Tips: Cashew butter is usually located near the grocery store's peanut butter. If you cannot find cashew butter, use almond butter. Just make sure it's not added sugar.

Ingredients

- 1 cup shredded green cabbage
- 1 cup chopped red cabbage
- 1 cup chopped carrot
- ¼ cup of water
- 3 tablespoons chopped shallots
- 1 tablespoon black sesame oil
- 1 tablespoon cashew butter
- ¼ teaspoon red pepper flakes, or add as needed
- ½ teaspoon ginger powder
- Provide hot water as needed
- 2 teaspoons roasted sesame

Preparations

1.In a medium-sized bowl, layer the green and red cabbage, then add carrots, water, and green onions.

2. In a blender, add sesame oil, cashew butter, red pepper flakes, and ginger powder. Mix until ingredients are emulsified. If the dressing is too thick, heat water next to a teaspoon

3. Pour the seasoning on the vegetables, add sesame, and eat.

____

Per Serving: Calories: 317 / Total Fat: 24.7G / Carbohydrate: 20.8G / Fiber: 6.6G / Protein: 7.2G

Sun-Dried Tomato Sauce

Servings: 4. Preparation time: 10 minutes

This uncooked sauce can be placed on salads or warmed and used with any Italian recipe in this book. Be sure to use sun-dried tomatoes without oil. Oil adds one ton of calories, so it's not on the Go list. If the dried tomatoes are hardened, immerse them in a little water before use.

Recipe Tips:: Ketchup is the key to the rich tomato flavor here. Don't miss it.

Ingredients

- 1 cup cherry tomatoes, halved
- ½ cup tightly packed sun-dried tomatoes
- 3 tablespoons coconut oil
- ⅓ cup of fresh basil
- 1 tbsp tomato sauce
- 1 teaspoon sea salt
- 1 teaspoon garlic powder

Preparations

1. In a food processor, mix cherry tomatoes, dried tomatoes, coconut oil, basil, ketchup, salt and garlic powder.

2. Pulse merge until desired consistency is reached.

____

Per Serving (1/2 cup): Calories: 132 / Total Fat: 12.2G / Carbohydrates: 6.1G / Fiber: 1.5G / Protein: 1.4G

Enchilada Sauce

Servings: 8. Preparation time: 5 minutes. Cooking time: 26 minutes

This sauce is so delicious that you want to dip everything. After tasting, you will never buy canned food again. Frozen so you have it on hand.

Recipe Tip: Before cooking, add a tablespoon of Dutch-processed cocoa powder to add flavor and reminiscent of a rat sauce.

Ingredients

- 2 tablespoons coconut oil
- 2 tablespoons coconut flour
- 2 tablespoons paprika
- 2 cups of water
- 1 can (8 ounces) tomato sauce
- 1 teaspoon garlic powder
- ½ teaspoon cumin
- ½ teaspoon onion powder
- ½ teaspoon sea salt
- ¼ teaspoon red pepper flakes

Preparations

1. In a medium hot pot over medium heat, heat coconut oil, coconut flour and paprika. Cook for one minute so that the flour does not eat raw.

2. Add water, tomato sauce, garlic powder, cumin, onion powder, salt and red pepper powder to taste. Bring the mixture to a boil for 25 minutes, stirring occasionally.

3. Servings: is warm.

____

Per Serving (½ cup): Calories: 68 / Total Fat: 3.6G / Carbohydrate: 8.3G / Fiber: 1.6G / Protein: 1.8G

Homemade Barbecue Sauce

Servings: 6. Preparation time: 5 minutes. Cooking time: 25 minutes

What is summer without barbecue? This sauce tastes great on grilled vegetables, but does not contain the sour sugars found in bottled sauce. Feel free to try this recipe and add fruit or spices to it. It will stay in the refrigerator for about a week.

Recipe Tips:: This is especially good when made from peaches or mango. Just add ¼ cup when cooking for a sweet fruity flavor.

Ingredients

- 2 cups of water
- 1 chopped onion
- 1 can (8 ounces) tomato sauce
- ¼ cup apple cider vinegar
- 2 teaspoons paprika
- 2 teaspoons paprika
- 1 packet stevia

Preparations

1. In a medium pot, combine water, onion, tomato sauce, apple cider vinegar, paprika, paprika, and stevia. Boil the ingredients.

2. Reduce heat and simmer for 20 minutes on low heat.

3. Use immediately, or cool and refrigerate in a closed container.

____

Per serving (2 tablespoons): Calories: 36 / Total Fat: 0.8G / Carbohydrates: 7G / Fiber: 2.3G / Protein: 1.3G

Championship Chili

Servings: 4. Preparation time: 5 minutes. Cooking time: 25 minutes

There is nothing better than watching a bowl of peppers. This version fuses all the hearty, familiar flavors together to form a healthy meal. Using germinated beans can help reduce alkalinity. Do two batches and freeze the remaining food (if any)! Make sure to use diced tomato and pasta sauce, which contains no sugar, meat or dairy products.

Recipe Tips: Fresh coriander and dried coriander have different flavors. If you don't have fresh food on hand, ignore it completely from the recipe.

Ingredients

- Cooking spray
- 1 small onion, chopped
- 1 cup diced red bell pepper
- 2 cloves of garlic, chopped
- 2 cups sprouted beans (see here), black, kidney or pinto beans
- 1 (14.5 ounces) tomatoes that can be diced
- 2 tablespoons homemade barbecue sauce (here)
- 1 (8 ounce) canned organic pasta sauce
- ¼ cup medium, medium or hot organic salsa

- ¼ cup organic fresh coriander
- Dash Paprika
- Dill Cumin

Preparations

1.Spray the medium-sized pot with a cooking spray. Place it on medium heat. Add onions and fry for 5 minutes, or until onions are soft and slightly caramelized.

2. Add bell pepper, garlic, germinated beans, tomatoes, homemade barbecue sauce, pasta sauce, salsa sauce, coriander, paprika and cumin. Stir and mix. Stew for 20 minutes.

3. Serve immediately.

Per Serving (1 cup): Calories: 101 / Total Fat: 2.7G / Carbohydrates: 18.5G / Fiber: 5.3G / Protein: 3.9G

Cilantro Salad Dressing

Servings: 12. Preparation time: 5 minutes

Each salad dressing recipe in this chapter is a simple variation of a theme: one apple cider vinegar, two coconut oils, with different flavorings. The good news is that you will soon master the habit of making your own salad dressings without feeling the need to buy expensive, salty, sour sauces in stores. Have fun and play with these recipes.

Recipe Tips: In this recipe, do not use dried coriander or parsley. The taste varies. Pick the freshest coriander and rinse. If you want, you can cut off the stem.

Ingredients

- ½ cup coconut oil
- ¼ cup apple cider vinegar
- ½ cup chopped fresh coriander
- 1 teaspoon freshly squeezed lemon juice
- ¼ teaspoon sea salt
- ½ packet stevia

Preparations

In a blender, add coconut oil, apple cider vinegar, parsley, lemon juice, salt and stevia. Mix until the cilantro is fully incorporated and the oil and vinegar are emulsified.

____

Per serving (2 tablespoons): Calories: 80 / Total Fat: 9.1G /
Carbohydrates: 0.1G / Fiber: 0.4G / Protein: 0.3G

Asian Citrus Dressing

Servings: 12. Preparation time: 5 minutes

This seasoning can be used with any Asian dish in this recipe. A bowl of quinoa and steamed vegetables are also great. You want to use ginger and minced garlic instead of fresh in this recipe. Otherwise, the taste is too sharp.

Recipe Tips: If you prefer the umami flavor of fresh ginger and garlic, be sure to use fresh ginger and garlic. Just grind them into a blender.

Ingredients

- ½ cup coconut oil
- ¼ cup apple cider vinegar
- 1 tablespoon freshly squeezed orange juice
- 1 tablespoon black sesame oil
- 3 tablespoons chopped shallots
- 2 teaspoons roasted sesame
- ½ teaspoon ginger powder
- ½ teaspoon garlic powder
- ¼ teaspoon sea salt
- ½ packet stevia

Preparations

1. In a blender, mix coconut oil, apple cider vinegar, orange juice, sesame oil, shallots, sesame, ginger, garlic powder, sea salt and stevia.

2. Mix until the ingredients are well mixed and the oil and vinegar are emulsified.

____

Per serving (2 tablespoons): Calories: 90 / Total Fat: 1.1G / Carbohydrates: 1.1G / Fiber: 1.4G / Protein: 0.9G

Avocado Salad Dressing

Servings: 12. Preparation time: 5 minutes

If you have avocados that you need to use, this is a great recipe. Choose soft foods for the best flavor. This fits well with the Mexican recipes in this book. It has a lot of flavors, so you don't need much flavor.

Recipe Tips: If you like spicy, add jalapenos when mixing.

Ingredients

- ½ cup coconut oil
- ¼ cup apple cider vinegar
- 1 avocado, peeled and pitted
- ¼ cup chopped fresh coriander
- 1 teaspoon freshly squeezed lemon juice
- 1 teaspoon garlic powder
- 1 teaspoon cumin
- 1 teaspoon onion powder
- ¼ teaspoon sea salt
- ½ packet stevia

Preparations

In a blender, mix coconut oil, apple cider vinegar, avocado, coriander, lime juice, garlic powder, cumin, onion powder, sea salt and stevia. Mix until all ingredients are well mixed and the oil and vinegar are emulsified.

____

Per serving (2 tablespoons): Calories: 101 / Total Fat: 10.8G / Carbohydrates: 1.2G / Fiber: 0.9G / Protein: 0.2G

But you can't adjust your pH The purpose of the alkaline diet is NOT to seek to increase blood pH. Yeah, that's Good. The aim of the alkaline diet is NOT to attempt to increase blood pH.

The entire aim of alkaline diet is to avoid the controlling body!

This is the biggest misunderstanding so-called experts have which dismiss the alkaline diet so quickly. We really haven't completed enough homework, because the fact is, they are making themselves seem like fools.

Acidic diet's True risk Your doctor and buddy are totally right, as the body can do anything it takes to control the blood pH (and other cell fluids 'pH). But what triggers the huge issues of an excessively acidic diet and lifestyle is the relentless need to do the controlling.

They are relieving the body from its need to control by living and drinking alkaline and hence the body thrives. Of note, it benefits (and definitely isn't a coincidence) that all alkaline products are often nutrient-dense, organic, natural, nutritious, high-water-content, healthy foods full of vitamins, minerals and phytonutrients, antioxidants, etc.

Is the Alkaline Diet a Bit Comfortable?

I digress a little bit so do you believe this is a coincidence? Acidic diets are nutrient-devoid, toxic, artery-coagulating, dead diets, sugary foods, trans-fats, processed foods, oxidizing foods and foods that add zero nutrients to our body.

Whereas the very reverse of alkaline products. There are no alkaline foods which damage the body.

Tell me a doctor or writer or acquaintance who does not believe that a balanced lifestyle is the following: – plenty of organic ingredients – consume plenty of herbs, low sugar fruits, grains, berries, salads, drinks, smoothies – workout every day – stay stress-free and prevent toxins – stop trans fats, carbohydrates, processed oils, fried meats, unhealthy snacks, takeaways, beer, cigarettes, popcorn, cookies, candy, ice cream etc.

They actually weren't developing in a body to deal with the lifestyle shifts that the new environment has brought us. We have not developed enough that we can cope with such acidic Regular Western diet of yeasts, carbohydrates, trans-fats, microwave dinners, fast snacks, pizzas, cookies, candy.

Our body was not built so that so much acid could be neutralized!

The human body produces its own acids (metabolic acids) and we have developed with a tiny acid buffering mechanism that can quickly neutralize this acid produced by the internal mechanisms and metabolism of our body. Nevertheless, the body goes into shock as we put extremely heavy acids on top of it all day long – actively struggling to maintain the pH of the blood and other fluids at a somewhat alkaline pH of 7.365.

That is where the acid diet harm happens We truly realize and accept why the body must hold the pH of 7.365 ALWAYS and our intention is not to alter it! The goal is to give the body the resources it wants, so that it is as simple as possible to sustain this pH. Bringing tons and loads of acid-forming products sends the body through a big tailspin and snowballs that are harmful.

Constant consumption in over-acid diets and an over-acid diet contribute to major long-term problems. The body must make all kinds of long-term concessions to your wellbeing to maintain your short-term safety while maintaining the pH of your cell fluids at 7.365.

Calcium is drawn from the bones, magnesium is taken from the skin, and yeasts, microbes, and microform overgrowths are extremely active in the digestive system-clogging the intestines and creating all kinds of problems.

The alkaline diet is not meant to alter this 7,365 – it is directed at strengthening the organism, removing the burden of an acidic lifestyle and providing the organism the strength it requires to survive.

And the explanation is this: The body should maintain the blood pH at a really small range similar to pH 7.365 Still. Your goal is NOT to alter it, it's to help the actions of the body to hold it there. The normal, conventional, Western diet is highly acidic, and eating such an acid diet places intense strain on the body to attempt and neutralize such acids and maintain the pH at the somewhat alkaline 7.365 point. The true harm to the body is caused not merely by eating such products, but the main damage is the body's inability to work significantly hard to neutralize the acids and maintain the pH at 7.365.

And the next time anyone asks you the alkaline diet is pointless, you know the reaction to that now. Let them keep reminding themselves there's no sense of consuming alkaline, so they will start to slurp their drink and enjoy their burger. I mean, what does it matter anyway – does the body still hold this pH correct? And why try to stay good.

I assume that's all right. I tried to make things as straightforward as possible, but you can ask them below if you have any questions at all!

KNOWS lemons both are acidic. Why would you tell them?

That's a really popular issue, and I get pretty good at addressing it in a friendly and easy way!

Essentially, it's just the impact the food has on the body after eaten, rather than the actual acidity or alkalinity. Lemons, though they lack citric acid, have a very small concentration of potassium, magnesium and sodium, which are highly alkaline minerals. These minerals have a highly alkalising body influence.

The explanation that doesn't function on oranges is that the orange's sugar level is so high that it cancels out the alkalising minerals and creates a rather acidifying impact on the body. This (unfortunately) is the same with nearly all fruits.

Can I have any fruit?

Unfortunately, the answer to this one is usually yes (a little) and no ... certainly don't think of fruit the way other people do ... fruit can be viewed as a treat, or 'emergency food.'

Better than a candy bar, indeed, but the fruit's sugar content does render it very acidifying. There are a limited amount of alkaline fruits that I consume a Lot of, but most of them you might know of (banana, strawberries, pineapple, etc.) are producing acid.

You just ought to stop as far as practicable any of the carbohydrates, if it's fructose, sucrose, glucose (anything that ends in -ose).

They do have the same effect on the body-sugar is sugar, no matter from where you receive it and it's packed with a ton of berries.

Although I know that fruit also comprises protein, minerals, phytonutrients and so on, the vast quantity of fruit sugar means that this is not a worthwhile trade off.

When you want to consume berries, aim to reduce it to one slice of in-season berries a day and preferably seek to supplement it with a little healthy fat and protein, because that will balance blood sugar because soon as you consume fructose.

The problem with Sugar (and a brief crash course about why an acid diet is too bad) Much as our body will do whatever it needs to maintain 37 degrees hot, it will go to equal measures to preserve a pH level of 7,365 for our inner cells, particularly the blood.

The current Western diet of beef, cheese, fizzy beverages, snacks, cookies, sweets, beer, soda, pizza, rice, toast, etc. has a dramatically acidic body influence. Such an acidic lifestyle places tremendous tension and pressure on the body as it has to fire-fight continuously to maintain the pH of 7.365.

Food not only sucks up a Large amount of our resources (remember how you felt after Christmas dinner or a big takeaway meal?) but it also utilizes the alkaline minerals (buffers) in our body including calcium, potassium, magnesium and sodium. It in effect gives way to too many unimaginable health issues.

Such acid-forming foods and drinks often contain yeasts, bacteria and mold in our blood. Furthermore, the acids produced and ingested throughout our western lifestyle often ferment the blood and produce harmful by-products, pollutants and alcohols and therefore further kill our internal climate.

Further acid produces further chemicals, the pH becomes reduced, the bacteria and yeast expand, becoming mold and a destructive cycle starts.

Moreover, these toxic microbes, yeast and mold literally feed on the nutrients you ingest! But not because of it! The waste products which they leave behind even serve as their fuel, implying rapid multiplication!

Therefore, it throws our body into chaos as we eat sugar. Consumption of sugar is like pouring fuel on a spark. This loop is accelerated easily, compounding the dilemma and increasing an excessive amount of tension on the body.

I've written about this before and there are a variety of issues and problems that sometimes surface, but the problem that pops up more frequently is this: However fruit sugar is special isn't it? Is fructose good, right?

NOTHING. Fat is fruit and it is fat. Wherever it emerges from it does not matter, it always plays havoc in the body's acid / alkaline equilibrium. If it's from fructose, sucrose, corn, honey or a slice of chocolate cake, the sugar has the same destructive impact even. How rapidly or gradually the body metabolizes various sugars will influence the energy rates (in terms of how often the peaks and troughs can match each other) but will not make much difference to the reality that the sugar ferments and activates such unhealthy microforms in precisely the same manner.

Not consuming berries, too! It is clear to see that sugar is extremely unhealthy and made of seeds. And fruit juice as it were? Sugar juice is very literally extremely processed sugar, new or not! Not without the fiber! It's the same question that's being compounded by twenty. DO NOT DRINK JUIZE Water!

Are there some fruit Okay?

A range of low-sugar vegetables is here, good for you! Tomato, pineapple, ginger, lime and grapefruit are all produced from alkalising and goodness. So when anyone wonders how alkalising lemons so limes would be, the answer is simple: it's the effect the food has on the body, not whether it's normal in its acid or alkaline condition. The alkalising effect of the reason lemons and limes is that they are not only abundant in water and low in sugar, but they also contain high concentrations of alkaline minerals (especially potassium).

What is better green beverage (powdered leaf supplement)?

1. Was the drink green sugar free? There are so many supposedly green beverages out there (especially on the high street), that contain sugar and sweeteners very foolishly. Where is the point?! Look out particularly for carob & stevia. Note that it needs 20 alkaline components to neutralize 1 component acid, and if your greens contain sugar than at best you'll end up with pH neutral … leaving your green beverage expensively meaningless.

2. Is the natural beverage safe of yeast, fungus and algae? Most greens often contain yeast, mushroom extracts and algae that I actually do not suggest and recognize that Dr Young has proven extremely acidifying.

Red beverages 1. MegaGreens: A nice, fresh mix of organic New Zealand grasses 2. PH Ion Green: Tasting much sweeter, but it does contain spirulina, and I use it sparingly. A ton of our clients enjoy this one 3 experience. Tony Robbins Pure Energy Greens: a very special green soda to try, but still powerful 4. SuperGreens: Then the original of course. Still packs a punch.

What supplements should you suggest It is always down to your own particular nutritional necessity, so I will certainly recommend consulting to a professional nutritionist before undertaking any big dietary improvements – but in my own experience and through my customers 'reviews I prescribe to every food plan the following four supplements as a strong cornerstone: Supplement Suggestions 1 Green Drink: Heavily alkalising, rich with high nutrients and extremely healthy for health, green beverages are a must for me. I can almost promise that if you start getting four green drinks a day you'll start enjoying the results nearly immediately. A rich source of chlorophyll, vitamins, minerals, enzymes and other nutrients – the greens infuse the body with extremely alkaline products to cleanse, neutralize acids and give the body an immense boost of strength.

2. An anti-inflammatory: my research has demonstrated that maintaining optimal wellbeing is a mixture of an alkaline, antioxidant-rich, anti-inflammatory diet and lifestyle, so with any of these three it is also really necessary to provide a protection net. The green drink & salts (see below) are extremely alkaline, the greens are abundant in antioxidants and the remedy that I'm going to list + the oils are anti-inflammatory ... And this is curcurmin, the solution. It more usually comes with a remedy based on turmeric (some can also involve ginger, and

piperine, a black pepper compound that deals with the bioavailability of curcurmin).

The most advantageous form of curcurmin supplement from my research and personal knowledge, is curcurmin phytosome.

Curcurmin has been researched widely and its effects-more than any other natural drug.

3. Omega & Coconut Oils: I firmly urge you to concentrate on the omega 3 and coconut oil you are consuming for better health, strength and wellness. Here's a rundown of the important information you want to get you started!

Omega 3: The main omega 3s are ALA, EPA, and DHA. The human body can not spontaneously produce omega 3, so we need to boost our diets. Hence, Omega 3 is the fat we most need. Experts suggest we take about 20- of omega 3 a day to function optimally. Eating simply, even when we eat fried fish and nuts every day, finds it difficult to do that. Particularly when a lot of foods (including fish and meat) are processed in a manner that makes them less nutritious than in the last few days.

O Short Chain Coconut Oil Tryglycerides (MCT): MCT is challenging to bring across since almost the other oils that we consume are long chain. As it is almost always fresh, we discuss coconut oil, it is incredibly resistant to heat, light and air (as opposed to all other oils) and it can be cooked with and still healthy and it tastes amazing! It's a saturated fat, of instance, but the notion that saturated fats are bad to us has been utterly demolished and saturated fats are too good for you!

These essential fatty acids (EFAs) are deemed required, because they are completely necessary for the body to function, but they can not be produced on their own. It relies on us to consume certain fats, like omega 3 and omega 6. These fats are so important that we would all eventually fail because we haven't consumed any of these EFAs even though we fully eliminated the bad fats from our diets. We simply can't live without those fats!

Do you or have ever suffered from any of the following: * Dry skin, acne, or skin disorders such as eczema, psoriasis, or rosecea * Constipation * Weight gain * Poor hygiene * Thin hair and hair loss * Sluggish nail growth * Liver and kidney depletion * Exhaustion * Sleep deficiency * Stomach issues * Intestinal issues, diarrhea, bloating * Asthma * Ineffective library output

4. Alkaline Minerals: The main determinant of how a material creates alkalines is the alkaline mineral quality. Minerals contain salt, magnesium, potassium, calcium, manganese, zinc etc. So the first four are the four major alkaline formations: salt, magnesium, potassium and calcium.

I firmly recommend that you find these minerals as a high quality nutrient (or supplementS), preferably in the form of bicarbonate.

The amount of research on the impact of sodium bicarbonate is enormous. That is evident.

Potassium is likewise no brainer. The potassium-sodium ratio is too essential for our western diet and has become too out of balance. The problem is not sodium at all, it's that: a) most people eat a ton of the processed, condensed, healthless sodium chloride (regular table salt) instead of the mineral-rich Himalayan / Celtic natural salt b) most people don't really eat enough potassium, which throws the ratio out of whack.

Slowing down too much of the food sodium also presents its own dangers. Sodium is required-it is an important mineral of alkaline origin. But you need to bring down the potassium!

Where do I get protein from?

It's a really good question, but in the wrong way I think it's ... So, I'm trying to get there. The first thing you need to ask yourself is: 'How much protein do I require? '. Simple query. Robert Young (pH Miracle) says that the average individual needs just over 20 g a day, but that naturally varies when you're working out or leading a busy life. Currently I'm hitting about 50g-100 g depending on my workout / exercise level, but certainly nowhere near the heights of other coaches who claim you should weigh at least 2 g per pound.

I suggest choosing your own amount within the range (20-100 g) you're satisfied with and instead determining where to get your protein from. When most people inquire about the alkaline diet, it's mainly out of fear because they're not having enough-although the most relevant issue is-what's your protein supply, i.e. make sure it's a good source!

I consume at least 50g-60 g of protein a day on an alkaline diet without any extra nutrients which are more than enough for the body to function, expand and develop. Newly embraced protein-rich foods such as chickpeas, quinoa, chia, beans, lentils, berries, nuts, etc., still exceed 80 g of this number.

Often, I'm currently incorporating an organic sprouted brown rice protein when I reach the crossfit and run really hard, but that's not important if you're not either working out or in a gym.

Should I lose weight (OR should I add weight?) The body is alkaline by definition, and weight increase is one of the more obvious indicators of being over-acid.

Your body will hang onto fat to protect your primary organs when you are over-acid, and you also can not consume the excess fat from the acids you eat. Before you start alkalising you shred through this fat quickly. Bulges and cellulite disappear quite surprisingly rapidly.

There's a interesting idea behind this, because if you think you're going to constantly consume tons of fresh, healthy vegetables, bananas, nuts, grains, good fats, etc. to remain completely hydrated when consuming zero carbs, trans-fats, chocolate, crisps, chips, drinks, etc. Equally, being underweight is an acid epidemic. Your obstructed, over-acid digestive tract prevents the body from consuming the food that you consume, leaving you weak and lean. You'll be filling up in all the right places and contributing fat to the body before you start alkalising.

How do I check my pH-why are my readings erroneous?

The pH check is a perfect way to chart your development. Still you have to do it right. Here's how: Checking 1 hour before or 2 hours after feeding is great technique. If you're measuring the saliva, attempting to cover the mouth with saliva and then drink it is a smart idea. This assists in killing any harmful bacteria that could be lingering. Should not seek or something else to wash your mouth out because that would actually document the alkalinity of the water / liquid you've just used.

Let any urine flow before checking for urine tests as this will provide more of an average reading.

It is always a safe practice to check 2-3 times a day and obtain an average, because the body has absorbed fluids for a lengthy period of time first thing throughout the morning and can participate throughout numerous processes and eliminate acid production from the body during the day (depending on operation and diet).

What the variations and differences?

The explanation why there is such a discrepancy in the urine and saliva readings is because a) the mouth is more prone to have acidic bacteria during the day (if you brush your teeth it may display very strong alkaline reading due to toothpaste and there is not much space around it) and b) that your urine is more of a representation of the processes the body undertakes to absorb ac.

Therefore, these are prone to variations. I will consider taking on an average of many readings in order to get a broader perspective of the development, rather than relying on each reading alone.

A reading from 6.75-7.0 + from everywhere is good for saliva because saliva appears to be somewhat more acidic. A somewhat higher pH rating of 7.5 onwards is better for the urine, but note that the urine will provide a more irregular reading due to the kidneyâ€TMs absorption of contaminants during the day.

So place all of that in context, anyone consuming a traditional Western diet will be more likely to have an average saliva pH of about 5.5-6.0. This does not sound any smaller, but it is important to note that the pH scale is logarithmic – implying that each phase is ten times logarithmic, i.e. 4.5 is 10 times more acidic than 5.5, which is 100 times more acidic than 6.5 and so on.

Checking your saliva or urine at pH would just offer you a general pattern. Sadly there is no method to assess the blood's EXACT pH by needing to perform a live blood examination. We will provide a clear example, though – but check, check, test and take the average and then observe that pattern over time, noting the impact that some dietary improvements will create.

What is the most alkalising vegetable?

Not exactly something you need to care about too much, but if you need to ask-I guess it's a wheatgrass-cucumber toss-up. So essentially here's my short and dirty list of foods to be targeted at if you choose to avoid super-alkalising: green grasses – like wheatgrass & barley grass Green leafy veg – like spinach, rocket & watercress Cucumbers Avocados Tomatoes Every other lettuce, vegetable or high water quality, low sugar diet!

Only imagine huge salad bowls and large veggie dishes!

Could I just get so alkaline?

Basically, indeed, you will of course get too alkaline. That can be very, very hard to accomplish! Your body continuously produces acids in its everyday life, which is why we need to concentrate on consuming alkaline 80/20 diets to further neutralize such acids. Through consuming and drinking acidly we naturally make it worse too.

So if we were to consume SO alkaline that the cells and body fluids were over 7.365 so the body would only balance that and bring you down down to the correct pH. When you were so acid, the impact on the body will be equivalent. So considering that 99 percent of us are too acid 99 percent of the time (although we're always walking so living as humans!), so I don't believe it will impact us that much, you will actually act pretty much the same as you are doing right now.